THE HEALING HERBS OF EDWARD BACH

THE
HEALING HERBS
OF
EDWARD BACH

A Practical Guide to Making the Remedies

JULIAN *&* MARTINE BARNARD

Bach Educational Programme

First published in Great Britain 1988
by Bach Educational Programme
P.O. Box 65, Hereford, HR2 0UW

British Library Cataloguing in Publication Data
Barnard, Julian
The Healing Herbs of Edward Bach
1. Medicine. Plant Remedies
I. Title II. Barnard, Martine
615'.32

ISBN 0 9506610 4 X

Typeset in Mergenthaler Sabon by Five Seasons Press, Hereford
Colour origination by Lawrence Allen Ltd, Weston-super-Mare
Printed in Great Britain by Butler & Tanner Ltd, Frome and London

Acknowledgements

Our sincere thanks are due to the people who have helped form this book and who have made it possible. Many of our friends and our family have given encouragement and advice and we are grateful, particularly to Mr and Mrs P.N.Barnard. Pam Bailey, Glenn Storhaug and Ron St John helped with editing; Nickie Murray gave some essential advice on finding the plants, so too did Elizabeth and David Beale; the Haigh family and our own children also helped us search for the flowers. Michelle Challifour advised on the pictures and Chris Adam took the photograph on the back cover. The photograph on page 31 is by Malcolm Murray, page 65 from the Harry Smith Horticultural Photographic Collection, page 67 from the A-Z Collection, page 159 by Erik Pelham—our thanks to them all. The setting is by Glenn Storhaug of Five Seasons Press: as always we appreciate your help, thank you.

Note

In the text all references to Bach's writings are given as page numbers in *Collected Writings of Edward Bach*, published by Bach Educational Programme, 1987. They appear as *[C.W., 00]*. The 'Indications' are from *The Twelve Healers & Other Remedies* and are annotated as *[Twelve Healers]*.

Contents

Preface

During the early 1960s Nora Weeks and Victor Bullen painstakingly compiled a book which gave information on the plants and trees used in the Bach remedies. This was published in 1964 entitled *The Bach Flower Remedies, Illustrations and Method of Preparation*. It had water colour drawings that could be used as an aid to identifying the flowers. It also contained explicit instructions on how to prepare the remedies themselves by the *sun method* and *boiling method*. These processes have no great mystique about them and were published by Dr Bach himself, in the 1930s, in every different edition of *The Twelve Healers*. Miss Weeks tells us (in the *Bach Remedy Newsletter*, January 1964) that Bach had always hoped for such a book to be published so that those who wished might prepare the remedy essences for themselves. As well as providing the necessary technical information it invited an appreciation of the beauty of nature and stimulated the interest in and love for wild flowers that was an integral part of Bach's work and his discovery of the remedies. Sadly this book was not reprinted after Miss Weeks' death in 1978 although it would have been a real tribute to her personal commitment to keep the work of Dr Bach clear and freely available.

Nora Weeks had been Bach's assistant for many years and was well aware of the moral principles that guided his work. It is tempting to spell out what these were. But anybody who is in doubt as to what Bach thought can read his own words. Both in his book *Heal Thyself* and in his other writings (see *Collected Writings of Edward Bach*) he repeats time and again his wish to share his understanding freely and to serve his fellows. It was in just such a spirit that the original illustrated book was published. As Nora Weeks put it, it was a privilege to fulfil what was Bach's wish. The book was also a 'grateful memorial' in his honour. We can but echo her words.

During the ten years since the death of Nora Weeks there has been a vastly increasing interest in the Bach remedies and a corresponding increase in the sale of the bottles of stock. The modest service providing people with Dr Bach's 'healing herbs' has become a privately-owned limited company with businesses selling the product throughout the world. Times change. However, it is still possible for each of us to return to the simplicity of Bach's original formula and to go into the fields and seek the remedies directly and for ourselves. It is, after all, the 'herbs of the field' that provide the actual healing force. So this book with its photographs and information on the plants carries an implicit invitation to go back to the original source and see again what it was that led Bach to his great discoveries.

The methods that Bach devised for making the remedies were very simple. They were intended to maintain contact with the vital healing forces of the plants. These forces have been variously investigated but they are not easily described, rather they are something to be sensed directly. For some people the most pertinent question to ask is whether these forces can be of help to us, and, of course, they can. But there is increasing awareness that we need to understand what is really happening rather than just accept blindly the medicine or the idea. We want to take an intelligent part in the process. An opportunity for that is supplied by the general philosophy of Bach's work. By thoroughly understanding the remedy states that he described we can come to an understanding of ourselves. However, our self-discovery can be greatly enhanced by an appreciation of what these actual plants are and why they represent the things that they do. There is a great deal more to this than 'keep taking the drops'!

Finding out about the remedy plants has been fascinating and instructive. If we started off with the thought that we simply wanted the information of Nora Weeks' book to be available again, we soon discovered that the process of learning about the plants in itself was healing and delightful. Bach found the remedies originally by walking and searching and the process can be recommended. There is no doubt that we spend too much time indoors both physically and mentally. Looking for these wonderful healing plants has provided a welcome prompt to look again to nature, not theoretically or at third hand but practically, in a direct way. 'In the presence of the way of Nature disease has no power': so Bach wrote in the introduction to *The Seven Helpers*. The way of nature is in the fields.

No doubt those who live in the cities will feel that they cannot so easily escape into a rural idyll to gaze at the trees. But that is not what is meant. In part the attraction of the Bach remedies is that they can bring something of the pure force of nature into our lives. To develop that and to enhance its effect we need only begin to be aware that the Oak remedy is made from Oak trees, like those in the park; that the common conker tree has the healing qualities of White Chestnut. It is surprising that we can have known about a remedy like Agrimony for many years without ever consciously connecting it to the weed that grows in the lane by the house. Some of these plants are becoming scarce it is true, and that is in part the reason why photographs have been provided: they offer an alternative way to perceive the flower and its healing virtue.

This book represents to us a point of departure rather than any kind of arrival. Studying these plants, or any others, begins with getting to know them and that is a continuing process. It has been helpful to learn which remedy plants grow in our area—incidently Nora Weeks commended this to people living abroad (*Bach Remedy Newsletter*, June 1966) so that they could make their own remedies locally. Then by visiting the plants we can observe their growing as well as contact the healing forces there. Many people have favourite places, favourite flowers or trees and subconsciously they draw strength from them. One old lady at the age of ninety-three used to sit and gaze at a Chestnut tree in the garden. She had a photograph taken so as to remember it in flower throughout the year; instinctively she sensed that the tree had some special meaning for her. To make such a process conscious does nothing to impair it. We actually achieve far more by directing our thoughts with conscious intention than by drifting into a mysterious and subliminal state: that is the positive message of Clematis!

We trust that readers will find their own way in this subject and draw their own best benefit as they may. The gifts of nature are free and they lead to freedom. We are trying our best to understand life and offer this in the spirit of fellowship. We hope that the you will feel encouraged to look for the flowers and see that these are living plants and trees as well as being the names given to remedy states. The process of making even one remedy essence for yourself brings a deepening awareness of these healing herbs. We would hope that the book will give encouragement and confidence to those who wish to try this. As Bach wrote in *The Seven Helpers*: 'In this system of healing everything may be done by the people themselves, even, if they like, to the finding of the plants and the making of the remedies.'

Julian and Martine Barnard
Herefordshire, March 1988

Dr Bach and his flower remedies

The life and work of Dr Edward Bach has been written about extensively in several books. However, the following brief account may be of help to readers who are not well acquainted with his story.

Edward Bach was born at Moseley, near Birmingham, in 1886 and trained as a doctor in London. For several years he worked investigating the role of bacteriology in chronic disease. His researches led him to recognize that there were clear personality types that related to the various patterns of ill health, irrespective of the physical symptoms being presented by the patient. Working with vaccine therapy and later with homœopathic principles, he moved towards the discovery of the flower remedies. These he felt could help to harmonize the emotional imbalances that he came to see as the real causes of physical illness.

By 1930 he was prepared to give up his successful medical practice in order to search for the plants and trees that came to be known as *The Twelve Healers & Other Remedies*. These are the flowers described in this book along with the actual text that Bach wrote to describe these Thirty-Eight Healing Remedies. Each flower was found to embody the positive and harmonizing force for a negative emotional state, be it fear, resentment or despair. In order to transfer this healing force to a patient Bach prepared essences from the flowers. This essence, diluted to some extent, could then be taken as a medicine. He found that as the negative moods changed so the person would return towards health.

The healing properties of the remedies were explained by Bach in terms of a philosophy of life that saw a person as much more than the outward physical body that is treated in conventional medicine. Illness, he suggested, was a message from our inner being calling for a change in our way of living and our mental outlook. The primary purpose of the flower remedies is to help us to change and bring us back to a genuinely happy experience of life. These remedies have been in use throughout the world in the years since Bach's death in 1936.

Introduction

As we are all well aware, the English countryside is changing. And what applies in Britain is also more or less true elsewhere. In the sixty or so years since Bach discovered his flower remedies parts of our rural landscape have been altered out of all recognition. The post-war urban sprawl of housing has consumed land with an astonishing appetite and many of the fields and lanes that Bach may have walked, in the home counties, have disappeared. Our farmers too have been encouraged to change things. Hedges have been uprooted, mixed farming has given way to vast acreages of single crops, insecticide sprays and weedkillers have eradicated whole populations. Then there are the single mishaps like the spread of Dutch Elm Disease that destroyed the trees that were perhaps the most typical of the English countryside, at least in the south. We know that the landscape has always been adapted by the changing population and by changes in agricultural practice but like all things in this century the pace has accelerated.

The conservation movement is concerned by all this change since it puts under pressure many species of plants, insects and animals. But in the context of Bach's work this general concern may take on a more particular meaning. The loss of all these natural colonies is more than a moral issue, more than an aesthetic affront. Just as we human beings are a subtle expression of divine creation, so too are the plants. They are imbued with meaning. They express a climate of forces that are essentially a part of us. They both reflect and create the way we feel and behave. At the physical level we can see our mutual relationship in the way that the land responds to human activity. The relationship does not have to be destructive, it can create a natural harmony, but when we dominate nature we create something ugly where before there was beauty. It is greed and nihilism that have formed the ugliness of our environment just as it is our love of life that makes it beautiful. If the flowers are being destroyed then a part of our soul consciousness is going too. This is because the flowers are an outward expression of particular patterns of life force, patterns that express themselves in us as thoughts and feelings.

The idea that a flower embodies a thought is not so new. It is implicit for instance in the medieval courtly love tradition that idealized the rose, in the herbalists' doctrine of signatures or in the sentimental associations of the Victorian 'language of flowers'. But the suggestion here is rather more than this. It is that many flowers have a particular quality that is an exact equivalent to a human emotion. Bach recognized this and found that the flowers of the Mimulus for example, were a positive representation of human fear. That is to say, he found that the human emotion of fear is counteracted by the Mimulus flower. It manifests outwardly what we might call courage. Likewise the Chicory flower with its perfect blue is a manifestation of love. We may choose to accept this more as a poetic truth, saying that the flowers are a metaphor for this human emotion. But the plants are more than a metaphor, they do actually represent a thought. They are the physical presence of a thought form.

Like all thought forms they are to some extent interactive. We can be influenced in the thought that they represent but we can also influence them by the force of the pattern that we represent. It is rather a cartoon joke to picture a plant shrivelling up when we look at it, but it does happen to some extent if the look carries a strongly negative charge. It is the opposite of green fingers! The strength of a collective thought pattern, however, is more than that of one individual. So a colony of plants can withstand greater pressures as well as exert a greater field of influence. Collectively too our thoughts are more powerful. It is as a society or group that we first imagine, then design and make, houses, roads, planes and plastic. Collectively we have allowed the great changes that have taken place in the countryside. In a general way this is true because our desire has been for an increasingly materialistic society. In specific terms the increase in certain emotional patterns has led to the retreat of some kinds of plant. The sensitive ones go first and those concerned with balance and discrimination. So the Water Violet is finding it difficult to survive, its quiet and privacy invaded as much by the roar of human self-seeking as by machinery and drainage schemes. Equally the Scleranthus with its qualities of decisiveness and discrimination is less in evidence: it cannot withstand the weedkillers and the chemical fertilizers. This is signalling a change in the mental outlook of our society as we lose the faculty of deciding between right and wrong, what is good for life and what is destructive. Even a remedy like Rock Water (for mental rigidity) is affected since the chemicals used in farming and industry seep into the groundwater and give rise to pollution. Both the cause and the effect are that we live increasingly by theories without reference to the impact that they have in reality.

If certain of the remedy plants are under threat we can equally observe that in some places other species are coming to take their place. It would be interesting to study the thoughts that these more dominant plants represent. When planting trees on a new housing estate there is often a policy of choosing fast-growing ornamental species like the Japanese Cherries rather than the more traditional hardwoods such as Walnut, Oak, or Beech. As farmers plough and reseed old meadows they not only destroy the weeds (like Mustard and Centaury) but plant the chosen grasses that will yield high volume for silage. The voracious goat mentality of today strips the land so that few wild plants survive but then, when the crop is raised (be it wheat, oil-seed rape, sheep or cattle), a single, strong species blankets the earth. There is little blending or subtlety in so much of our contemporary thinking.

All of this has an effect upon the consciousness of the earth and it is this consciousness that gives rise to the thought forms of plant and tree. We are a part of it ourselves and respond to its call. Conservation and ecology are a response to the earth's need for balance. So too are Bach's discovery of the flower remedies, for if we understand how the plants can help us we will better recognize how we can live so as to help them. We will appreciate the way that all living things interrelate. As a subject of study this has a long way to go. We may know some of the reasons why a plant grows in certain physical conditions but as yet there is little concern for why it exists in its own terms. Those who seek to attune themselves to individual plants do learn more of their secrets and this in turn is offering a new vision of the planet's life. Whether we choose to describe this in terms of plant devas and angelic beings is not really very important, for there is a genuine attempt to recognize the guiding forces of creation and to see how they work in life. As we learn about them we may hope to live and work with cooperation rather than conflict. The results will become apparent in the world around us as these forces will help to change the consciousness of those who are responsible for the well-being of the earth.

In the past it has been the practice for specialists to do research and then publish their findings, in the manner of explorers giving an account of a new land to those who stayed at home. But this is a journey of discovery that we all need to take, individually and together. We shall learn most by making contact with the land and the plants ourselves not just by taking somebody else's word for the experience. There is no definite way in which this is to be done and our own experience will guide us, as will the silent teacher of our inner being. This is clearly the way that Bach approached the subject, as we can tell from his writings. What we learn then will be be in accordance with what we need to know so that we can better fulfil our life's purpose. This is consistent with Bach's understanding of how we can achieve health by using flower remedies—always the inner directive from the soul leads us towards experiences that are necessary for us and that will lead us to be happy in life.

The process of coming to meet the plants has been called attunement: we learn to listen to the tuning vibration of the plant. Inevitably this has a rather personal quality to it. The description of what we experience individually can sometimes appear vague or even fanciful to those who are out of sympathy. But it can be used to inform and vitalize a more objective approach that is based upon outward observation. We need to feel the living forces of nature as well as see them as external phenomena. That way we can realize how they are part of us and we of them. Ideally there is a balance between the inner and outer experience so that we can come to a better understanding of what these plants are and how they each express their particular nature.

There is much to learn in just finding the remedy plants and observing them. At first it may be difficult to identify an individual flower and many hours can be spent in fruitless searching. But, as we see one and then another, we recognize the gesture of the remedy and begin to see with the inner eye the quality of it. We begin to know the feeling of how and where it grows and sense the reason for its being there; equally we can recognize why it will not be found elsewhere. In a similar way it is helpful to see how the flowers compare with each other—the flower of Cherry Plum may appear a little like Crab Apple, for instance, though its growth and manner of flowering mark it off as quite different. The colour of these flowers points to something of their quality as remedies. We also can see them as a part of a far greater pattern in the landscape of colour as it changes through the seasons. This does not follow exactly the spectral sequence but the year starts with white, leads on through yellow (and red) to blue and purple.

The individual colours play a large part in the subtle nature of the remedy flowers. Blue flowers like Cerato, for instance, express a more receptive feeling: the yellow or red flowers of Mimulus or Elm are more dynamic. This polarity of colour can be seen as the blue darkness of space into which the yellow sunlight shines. Where they meet on the surface of the earth, green leaves of the plant kingdom result. So too, the green of spring is a meeting of the darkness of winter with the summer light. This can be seen as significant in the green flower remedies like Scleranthus and Wild Oat which are concerned with balance, the balance that mediates between light and dark, above and below. Each individual flower is coloured that way for a reason. So the plant remedies for fear have a dynamic colour that projects a bright strength. The exception is the grey Aspen, although parts of the flower can be seen to be deep red when examined closely.

The way the flowers present themselves at different levels between the earth and sky is also significant. Some plants hug the ground (like Scleranthus), some try to gain height on frail stems (Wild Oat), others are held aloft by mighty trunks and branches (Sweet Chestnut). In a similar way there is a difference between the dangling catkin (Aspen), the flower that faces out horizontally (Chicory) and the erect flowerhead that holds the petals out to face the sun (Star of Bethlehem). The size, shape and colour of the flower, the locality, the soil, the community of other plants, the time of flowering, all these things have a meaning and can be read as more than the facts of physical information. Observing these things will help us better to understand the flowers that we are working with and help us to be more consciously attuned to nature altogether. Then, when we come to make a remedy (or even pick a lettuce come to that), we will be more sensitive, aware and awake to what is happening.

How to use this book

It is an important part of the function of this book that it provides the necessary technical information for those who wish to make remedies for themselves. But it is felt that there are other possibilities that can be mentioned here that may be of use. People who use a pendulum to dowse for an appropriate remedy can use the photographs in the book for diagnosis. And this could be done by just looking at the pictures: we will be attracted intuitively to the flowers that have significance for us. The pictures are intended to represent the feeling of the remedy as well as give the reader a copybook illustration and by selecting a remedy visually we may be able to come closer to the original healing force of the flower. The photographs could equally be used for treatment, as contemplating the image will offer another way to attunement. However, they are not likely to be as beneficial as going out to find the plant or tree itself. By including the text from Bach's *Twelve Healers & Other Remedies* it is possible to use the book for more conventional diagnosis. The affirmations, all chosen from Bach's own writings will offer a positive thought for use in meditation. This can strengthen us by bringing into focus that which we wish to become, that which we are moving towards.

The table of flowering times may assist us in planning a year of observation and discovery. It is really helpful to take the time to learn about particular flowers before going off to make a remedy. It will be advisable to obtain some standard textbook on plants and trees (see bibliography (p.175) that can supplement the general notes on identification that have been provided here. It is extremely important to get the identification right; mistakes are easily made. This plea for accuracy was made directly by the information office of the Royal Botanic Gardens at Kew. They also pointed out that whilst there are a great many Oak and Beech trees which will not miss the odd few flowers, some of the remedy species are becoming scarce. It is counter to the spirit of Bach's work and all that it stands for if we thoughtlessly take plants and flowers that need our protection and care. This is obvious and we all know it but it must be fairly stated again: please do not pick flowers if that will leave the colony of plants weakened. By the same token we should always take the book to the flower rather than the other way around. It may be a nuisance to carry books for identification when we are out looking for flowers, but there are several remedies that do require the utmost care to ensure that the plants are really the ones selected by Dr Bach.

Flowering periods for the plants

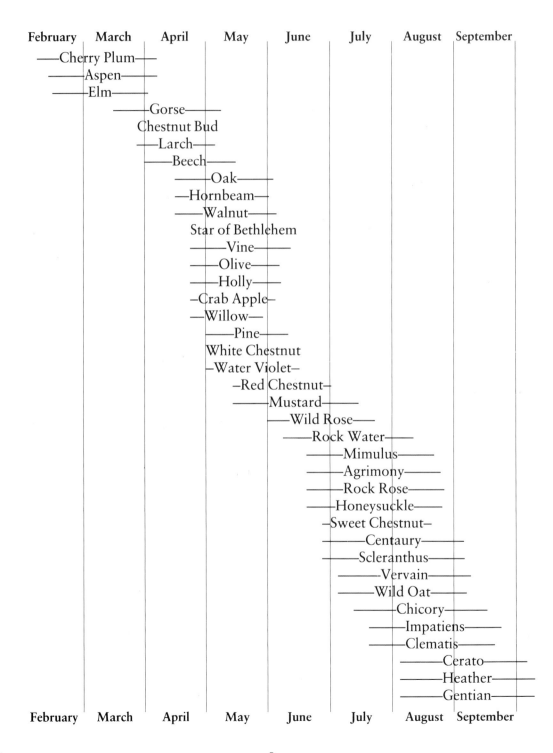

February | March | April | May | June | July | August | September

——Cherry Plum——
———Aspen———
——Elm——
———Gorse——
Chestnut Bud
——Larch——
——Beech——
——Oak——
——Hornbeam——
——Walnut——
Star of Bethlehem
——Vine——
——Olive——
——Holly——
—Crab Apple—
——Willow——
——Pine——
White Chestnut
—Water Violet—
—Red Chestnut—
——Mustard——
——Wild Rose——
——Rock Water——
——Mimulus——
——Agrimony——
——Rock Rose——
——Honeysuckle——
—Sweet Chestnut—
——Centaury——
——Scleranthus——
——Vervain——
——Wild Oat——
——Chicory——
——Impatiens——
——Clematis——
——Cerato——
——Heather——
——Gentian——

February | March | April | May | June | July | August | September

Preparing flower essences

When Dr Bach set out to make an essence he prepared himself beforehand so that he was in a receptive and harmonious state. Then he was able to work with the healing forces of nature that were to be brought into focus in the remedy. He would take a bath, wear clean clothes, a white gown and, so we might guess, he also prepared himself mentally by a form of meditation. Making a flower remedy calls for our best endeavour in all respects whatever way we choose to approach the process for ourselves. The more we strive to understand what is involved the better we shall be able to see what exactly is appropriate. Having found, on a previous occasion, a place where the plants or trees grow particularly well, we should choose a fine day for making the remedy and have everything ready. We may need ladders for the trees if the flowers are out of reach or a walking stick to hook a branch. Secateurs and scissors may be required or another chosen cutting implement. We may need permission from the landowner. Whether the remedy is made by the sun method or whether it is a 'boiler', the jugs, bottles, water and brandy must all be prepared before we start.

The Flowers – It is important to choose a location where these are growing naturally. Whenever possible they should be in the wild, in a place where they are not interfered with by animals or people, and where the earth forces are strong and unpolluted by motorways, power stations and the like. It is apparent that many of the remedy trees and plants no longer grow in the same clear and healthy conditions that existed in Bach's time. There are physical and metaphysical forces that have weakened and distorted the land and the flowers. Where the natural balance has been maintained there the remedy will be strongest. With those trees and shrubs that are likely to have been planted such as Red Chestnut, Walnut or Cerato we can find a place where the estate, farm or garden is sensitively cared for. When preparing a remedy use only those flowers that are in perfect bloom and select from several different plants or trees at the same location. Make doubly sure that this is the correct flower.

Equipment – A jug and funnel will be needed, the glass bowl or saucepan (according to which method is being used) and a bottle for storing the essence. These all need to be completely clean. They should be sterilized by boiling for twenty minutes in a large saucepan, wiped dry and wrapped in a clean cloth. A bottle of the purest water available is required (not distilled water) and a quantity of pure brandy to preserve the essence. Filter papers will be needed to strain the essences prepared by boiling.

Sun Method – Start making the essence before nine o'clock in the morning on a clear, bright, sunny day when there are no clouds in the sky. Take a thin glass bowl about 300ml or half pint size (not the oven-proof type) and fill it with pure water, preferably from a local spring. Pick the blooms from the plant and float them immediately on to the water. It may help if someone holds the bowl beneath the flower stems; alternatively carry the flowers on a broad leaf to avoid any contact with the hand. Cover the surface of the bowl and then top up the water if necessary. Leave it in the sunshine alongside the remedy plants for three to four hours, or less if the blooms show signs of fading. If the sun becomes clouded during this time the remedy should be abandoned. Avoid letting shadows fall across the bowl, whether your own or from plants and grasses. When they have given up their healing strength the flowers should be lifted out from the bowl using a twig of the plant rather than fingers. The essence is then poured into a clean, empty bottle so that an equal volume of brandy may be added as a preservative. It may be easiest to use the brandy bottle itself since it should be sterile, mixing the brandy half and half with the essence. It is up to you how much essence you choose to keep. When the remedy has been prepared you will sense the vitality and see that the water has been subtly changed.

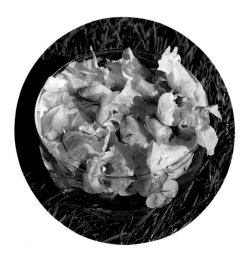

Boiling Method – Make the remedy on a bright day picking the flowers before nine o'clock in the morning. Take a clean enamel saucepan (aluminium should be avoided, stainless steel could be used but enamel is best), and three-quarters fill it with the flowers and stems. These need to be about 15cm long depending on the width of the pan. Put the lid on and take the saucepan home without delay. Then cover the flowers and twigs with two pints (1.13 litres) of pure water and put the saucepan on to boil, *without the lid on*. Simmer for thirty minutes using a twig of the plant to press the contents down if necessary. When the time is up, replace the lid and put the pan outside to cool. When it is cold the essence should be filtered. It may be helpful to remove the twigs first, again using a piece of the plant and not fingers. After filtering pour the essence into a bottle half and half with brandy. The boiling method prepares a large volume of essence and not all of it need be kept. It is interesting to taste a glassful on its own. The saucepan must be thoroughly cleaned and then boiled, along with the other utensils, and stored for future use.

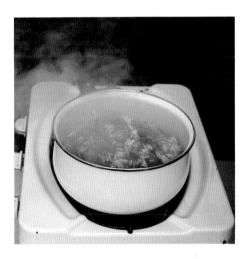

Essence : Stock : Medicine – When the essence is prepared and bottled it should be labelled. Provided it is kept free from physical and metaphysical interference it will retain its potency. Stock may be prepared by putting two drops of essence into a small (30ml) bottle filled with pure brandy. From such stock a chosen combination of remedies may be made up to medicine strength by placing two drops of each stock into a small bottle of water and brandy. Dosage is then four drops of this four times a day. Alternatively the two drops of stock may be put into a glass of water and sipped.

It is worth remembering that one small bowl of essence prepared by the sun method will supply enough of the remedy stock for thousands of people. The sum is revealing: a small glass bowl containing 300ml (half a pint) will contain approximately 3,600 drops. With the brandy this will make 7,200 drops of the essence. It takes two drops of this essence to potentize a 30ml stock bottle of brandy. So the essence will prepare about 3,600 bottles of stock. Each 30ml bottle of stock can prepare 180 bottles of medicine strength remedy. So we could obtain more than half a million bottles at the treatment strength (each bottle being sufficient for one person for three weeks) from the one rather small bowl of essence. This is really low cost medicine.

THE
THIRTY-EIGHT
HEALING REMEDIES

AGRIMONY

AFFIRMATION

The lesson of this plant is to enable you to hold peace in the presence of all trials and difficulties until no one has the power to cause you irritation.

[C.W., 105]

INDICATION

The jovial, cheerful, humorous people who love peace and are distressed by argument or quarrel, to avoid which they will agree to give up much.

Though generally they have troubles and are tormented and restless and worried in mind or in body, they hide their cares behind their humour and jesting and are considered very good friends to know. They often take alcohol or drugs in excess, to stimulate themselves and help themselves bear their trials with cheerfulness.

[Twelve Healers]

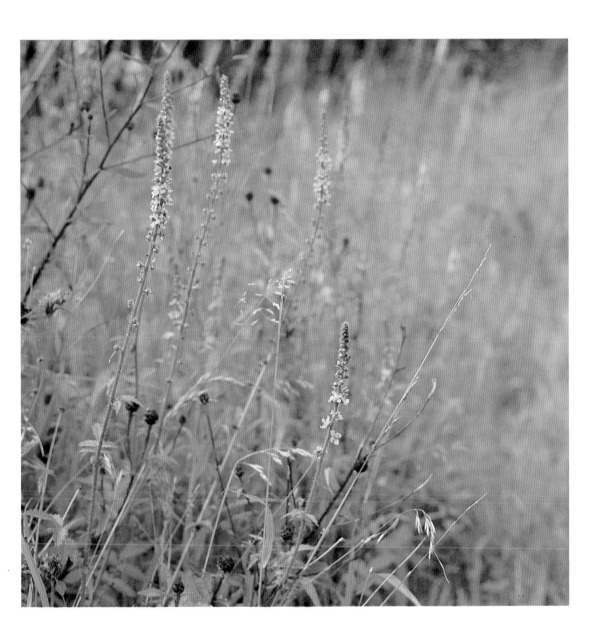

Agrimony *Agrimonia eupatoria*

Agrimony was one of the original *Twelve Healers*, found by Dr Bach in the summer of 1930 when he was staying in Norfolk. It is a flower that can bring calm to those who are inwardly anxious and in torment yet make a show of jollity. Traditonally a liver herb it is still used as a tonic tea especially in France. The liver is the seat of emotion and this remedy works to clear suppressed and obstructed emotions bringing peace and stillness. It also helps us to integrate and learn from experiences (often painful ones) that otherwise might be left in the depth of our being while we try to play across the surface of life. This is a remedy plant that brings a true depth and perspective, a discernment and acceptance of the varying qualities and expressions of our emotional life.

Describing 'that beautiful plant Agrimony...with its church-like spire, and its seeds like bells', Bach says it will bring 'the peace that passeth all understanding' *[C.W., 105]*. One of the colloquial names for Agrimony is Church Steeples— like the spire it aspires to the higher realm, growing straight upwards from a small rosette of base leaves. The pattern of its growth reflects its nature: the single purpose that even a flower can have to grow straight towards the source of life. With its deep tentacle roots and its single spire of flowers it is a witness to the one direction of growth that can bring peace and resolve conflicts.

Locality – Agrimony is a perennial found on hedge banks and roadside verges, in grassland and waste places; it often grows on chalk where the thin soil makes for shorter grass and so less competition. It will not tolerate acid soils or more than slight shade. It is common throughout the whole of southern England wherever mowing, grazing or spraying has left plants an opportunity to grow. It becomes increasingly scarce going north.

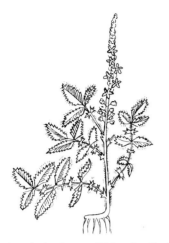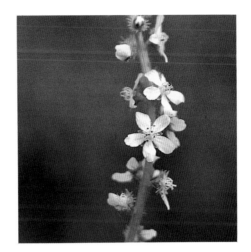

Left: the whole plant.   *Right: detail of the flowers.*

Identification – Agrimony should be easy to find because the spike of yellow flowers (a raceme) stands out above the surrounding grasses. Young plants make a single spike of 30-50 cm while a mature specimen reaches up to nearer a metre with a few branching stems. Along the tapering flower spikes the buds open progressively from the bottom revealing small five-petalled yellow flowers of 5-8mm on short stems. The lower flowers turn to fruits while those above are still in bud. The growing tip of the plant often droops slightly. The fruits have small hooks that catch on to the fur of animals or clothes of passers by.

The leaves are similar to some other plants being pinnate (divided up into pairs of leaflets along a mid-rib) and dark green. In spring they resemble such leaves as those of Meadowsweet, but these are smooth while in Agrimony the stem and leaves are hairy. A possible resemblance might be found in the Mullein, another flowering spike of yellow five-petalled flowers, but Mullein is larger, the leaves are single, oval and pointed. One related variant is *A. odorata* (or *A. procera*) which is said to be larger and more scented. The sub-division is not followed by all authorities and need not concern us.

Flowering Period – from June through to August. It is a flower of high summer.

Preparation – Agrimony is prepared using the sun method (see p.20). Select from several different plants that are well in flower. Cut the stems above any faded blooms or seeds that are forming and without too many buds at the top. It is best to pick from young plants early in the season. Do not remove individual blooms but cover the bowl with these flowering stalks. Choose a place where many plants grow together and set the bowl in their midst but where no shadows will fall on to the surface.

ASPEN

AFFIRMATION

The development of Love brings us to the realization of Unity, of the truth that one and all of us are of the One Great Creation.

The cause of all our troubles is self and separateness, and this vanishes as soon as Love and the knowledge of the great Unity become part of our natures.

[C.W., 155]

INDICATION

Vague unknown fears, for which there can be given no explanation, no reason.

Yet the patient may be terrified of something terrible going to happen, he knows not what.

These vague unexplainable fears may haunt by night or day.

Sufferers are often afraid to tell their trouble to others.

[Twelve Healers]

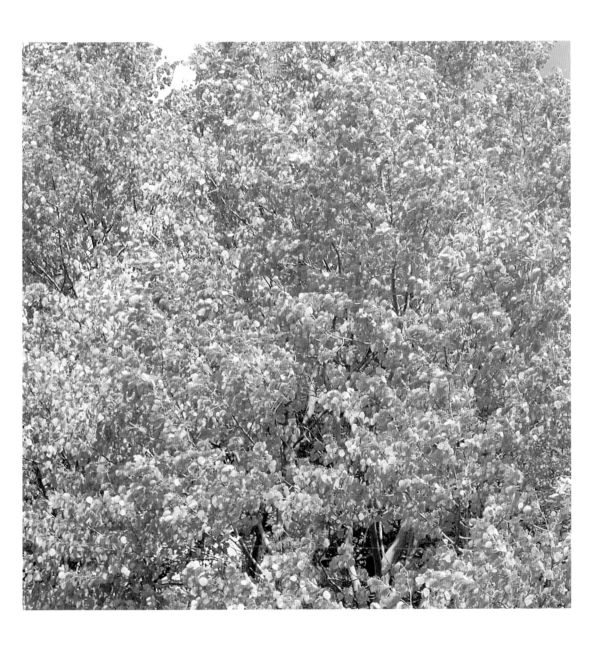

Aspen *Populus tremula*

The Aspen trembles, even on still days when there is barely a breath of wind the leaves may quiver as if some secret fear grips the tree. Why? One reason would be the flattened stalks of the leaf. Christian folklore says that this was the tree used to make the cross of the crucifixion and so the tree trembles in anguish at the memory. To Bach the tree was speaking of its nature, and it presents the picture of a hidden, unknown fear. This is the remedy state for Aspen. He describes it as a fear of 'vague unaccountable things which cannot be explained. As if something dreadful is going to happen, without any idea as to what it might be' [C.W., 8]. The remedy made from Aspen flowers brings a confidence and courage that calms such fear, that stills the troubled soul. It is a state of mind Bach says that can afflict people particularly when they are on the path of trying 'to do a little good on our journey through the world' [C.W., 23]. We may have the courage to overcome physical fears but as we try to live more by the moral standards of the inner world so we are the more likely to meet the fears that derive from that world too.

The tree was one of the second nineteen of the Thirty-Eight Remedies that Bach discovered. These were all found in 1935 in the region around Sotwell where he was living. As it begins to flower in the cold damp days of early spring it is one of the first remedies to be seen in the annual cycle. Writing in July 1935 Bach commented that 'there is no doubt that these new remedies act on a different plane to the old. They are more spiritualized and help us to develop that inner great self in all of us which has the power to overcome all fears, all difficulties, all worries, all disease.' [C.W., 23]. Aspen brings to earth some of the forces that are there, unknown, in the future for all of us. We feel them in the prospect of death and what lies beyond this mundane reality, in the prospect of a reality beyond our ordinary senses.

Locality – Aspen is found throughout Britain on poor soils and in damp woodland, more in the north and west as it is a pioneer species. Its tendency to sucker creates small thickets.

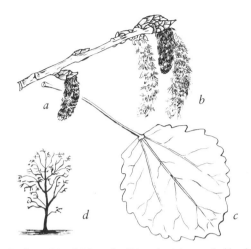
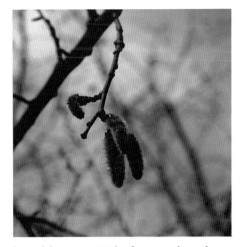

Left: catkins (a) female, (b) male; (c) rounded leaf, (d) outline of the tree. **Right:** *flowering branches.*

Identification – Aspen is a small tree (up to about 15m) being slightly built, unlike the great Black Poplar to which it is related. The grey catkins appear before the leaves. Other Poplars have more red in the flowers although Grey Poplar (which may be a hybrid between White Poplar and Aspen) is very similar. The Grey Poplar (*P. canescans*), however, is a larger tree (30m) with a lobed leaf. Male and female Aspen flowers are found on the same tree. The males are grey and have red anthers that are yellow with pollen when in full flower, some 5-10cm long. The females are smaller and green-grey. In May these cast seeds that are carried in white down that drifts in the wind like other Poplars. The bark is smooth and a luminous silvery green, the twigs are slender and the winter buds are bright brown. The leaves have a flattened stalk (which induces the trembling) and are smooth and hairless with a rounded form and a scalloped edge. Other Poplars have either whitish wool on the underside of the leaf (*P. canescans*) or an even fine-toothed leaf (*P. tremuloides*). It will be helpful to identify Aspen in the summer: examine the leaves.

Flowering Period – from February to early April.

Preparation – Aspen is prepared by the boiling method (see p.20). Both male and female flowers are used. Gather them from several trees where Aspens are growing in a thicket. Cut pieces 15cm or so with leaf buds and clusters of flowers.

BEECH

That we never criticise nor condemn the thoughts, the opinions, the ideas of others; ever remembering that all humanity are God's children, each striving in his own way to find the Glory of his Father.

[C.W., 32]

For those who feel the need to see more good and beauty in all that surrounds them. And, although much appears to be wrong, to have the ability to see the good growing within. So as to be able to be more tolerant, lenient and understanding of the different way each individual and all things are working to their own final perfection.

[Twelve Healers]

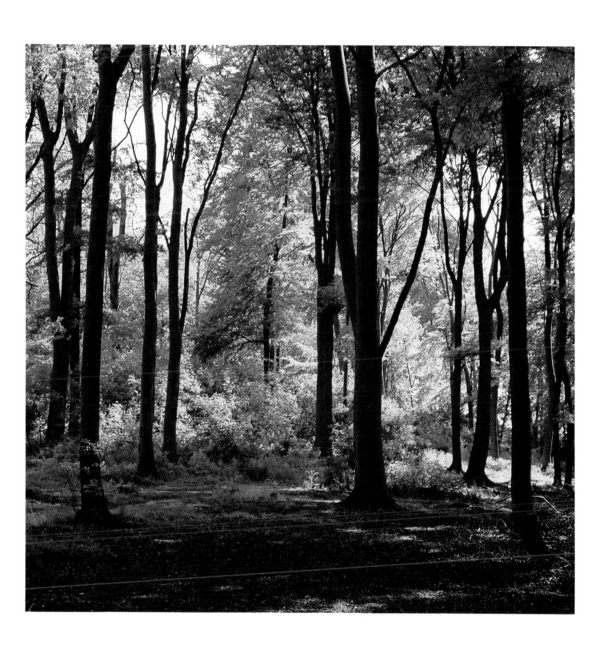

Beech *Fagus sylvatica*

What could be more beautiful than the sun shining through the spring leaves in a Beech wood? What is lovelier than the autumn colours of the Beech trees on the Chiltern Hills? These elegant woodlands provided Bach with a remedy for the state of mind that is critical, intolerant and fault-finding. It is true that the Beech is a refined and almost perfect tree. It has a smooth bark with a hard-grained and knot-free wood which can be polished to a superb finish; the young leaves covered with soft hair and minutely pleated, the purest pale translucent green, are a miracle of precision and fineness. So too, the mind that sees only the crooked hem, a speck of dirt and the imperfections of life: it too is precise and highly refined. But like the Beech tree too much refinement brings a critical and intolerant outlook if it develops negatively. In these woods no other shrubs or trees are tolerated; they are excluded by a carpet of dead leaves and the dense canopy of the tree tops which allows little rain or light to filter through. Once Beeches have come to dominance they reign supreme.

The critical mind finds fault with others to protect itself. Intolerance is used to give a sense of security. In Beech woods the trees are actually weak and shallow rooted, falling in storm winds if once they are exposed by woodland clearance. The Beech state of mind betrays a fear of life as much as a feeling of superiority. So the positive quality that this tree can bring is a vision of beauty that can see beauty in others, a way of perceiving the virtue in all things, a loving acceptance of life with all its imperfections and crumpled realities. In this positive state we can see that there are standards of behaviour other than our own that may be equally valid and have an equal right to exist; each being is working to perfection in the way of its own nature. Not all trees have to grow like the Beech, thanks be!

Locality – Beeches are found throughout Britain growing on a variety of soils. They are especially characteristic of chalk landscape preferring the well-drained conditions. Ancient Beech forests are generally found in the south of England.

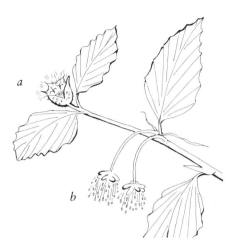
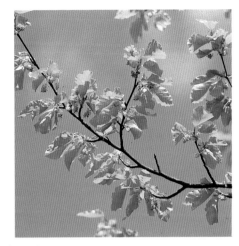

Left: flowers (a) female, (b) male.   ***Right:** a flowering branch.*

Identification – Beech is a native British tree growing to over 30m with a smooth grey bark. In woodland they often have no low branches though solitary trees will grow to a complete and balanced form with branches offering leaves for all available light. Leaf buds are long and slender on opposite spurs. Flowers form soon after the leaves appear with male and female on the same tree. The females mature a few days before the males to ensure cross pollination from a neighbouring tree. They are seen as a reddish crown of bristly 'mast' which hardens to protect the nut. The male flowers hang beneath the branch on slender stalks like clustering earrings. They swing in the wind and so release pollen. The Copper Beech and Weeping Beech are both ornamental derivatives of *F. sylvatica* and they are not the true form.

Flowering Period – April and May, soon after the leaf appears. The male flowers open as fluffy balls when ready.

Preparation – Beech is prepared by the boiling method (see p.20). Choose a place where the branches are accessible at the edge of a wood and pick from several different trees. Both male and female flowers are used. The females are mostly on the tips of the branches. Cut the twigs about 15cm to fit the saucepan.

CENTAURY

Centaury, that grows in our pastures, will help you to find your real self, so that you may become an active, positive worker instead of a passive agent.
[C.W., 106]

INDICATION

Kind, quiet, gentle people who are over-anxious to serve others. They overtax their strength in their endeavours.

    Their wish so grows upon them that they become more servants than willing helpers. Their good nature leads them to do more than their own share of work, and in so doing they may neglect their own particular mission in life.
[Twelve Healers]

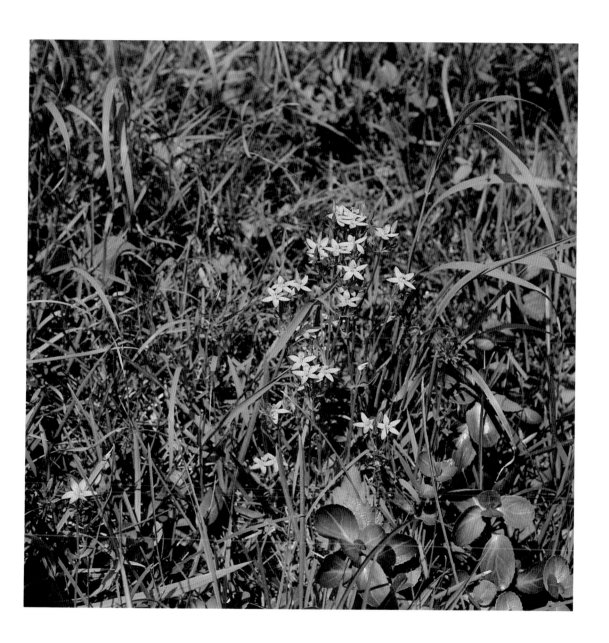

Centaury *Centaurium erythaea*

Meekness has been seen as a virtue. To be humble, mild and inoffensive is often thought to be praiseworthy, to be accepting and longsuffering is looked upon as being good—as Paul said to the early Christians of Colossus: 'Put on then as God's chosen ones, holy and beloved, compassion, kindness, lowliness, meekness and patience....' Yet while modesty may be preferred to pride there are times when meekness can go too far and instead of being a manifestation of true soul development it becomes a signal of weakness and lack of purpose. A slave may be meek and avoid the call to freedom; the bully only becomes strong because the weak do not assert themselves. Since this is a primary condition of human experience it is represented as one of the original Twelve Healers in the plant that Bach saw as bringing strength: Centaury. With its modest, unassuming beauty, it offers a purposeful clarity to the overhumble and weak.

Centaury grows strongly where many other flowers cannot find a footing, in dry thin soils. Its pale green leaves and soft pink flowers are like no other. To the casual glance they appear to be of little consequence and are easily overlooked in amongst the grasses; but look again and they are bright stars of radiance, the vibration of their delicate colour making others look crude, the simple perfection of their tiny florets calling to another world of gentle delicacy. Not languid, nor fay but strong, clear and bright. Bach did not expect the servant to become the master nor the downtrodden to become the bullies: this flower is not there to create an opposite but a real strength of individuality. Then will there be a true compassion that feels sympathy and the willingness to help without a losing of the self in servitude—a service of love among equals.

Locality – Centaury grows throughout Britain, except Scotland, in open grassland. It prefers dry soil, sometimes sand (there are various coastal varieties like *C. littorale* and *C. scilloides*); it grows commonly on chalklands, but not on acid soils. It will not tolerate shade. In longer grass it grows taller and more leggy, and conversely smaller in short grass.

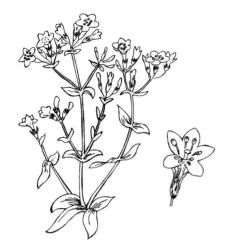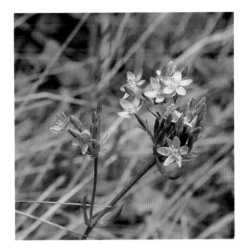

Left: structure of the plant.   ***Right:*** *detail of the flowers.*

Identification – Centaury is one of the family of Gentians of which there are several hundred throughout the world. There are about half a dozen different Centauries, all annuals. The Common Centaury (*C. erythaea* or *C. umbellatum*), which is the one to use, is easily distinguished from other local variants. Anything from 5-50 cm tall it grows on erect green stems from a rosette of leaves. There are a few small elliptical leaves, ribbed and smooth, without stalks, in opposite pairs on the branching stems. The pale pink flowers are five-petalled and held in clusters (umbels). Each one opens separately in warm sunshine before midday and closes again towards evening. Other varieties such as *C. pulchellum* lack the rosette of base leaves, are darker pink and have flowers individually stalked. Reference to a good *Flora* will point to exact identification.

Flowering Period – From June to September.

Preparation – Centaury is prepared by the sun method (see p.20). Find a place where a strong colony has grown up placing the bowl in the midst. Pick the open flowers only, so as to cover completely the surface of the water.

CERATO

Cerato will help you to find your individuality, your personality, and, freed from outside influences, enable you to use the great gift of wisdom that you possess for the good of mankind.

[C.W., 108]

Those who have not sufficient confidence in themselves to make their own decisions.

They constantly seek advice from others, and are often misguided.

[Twelve Healers]

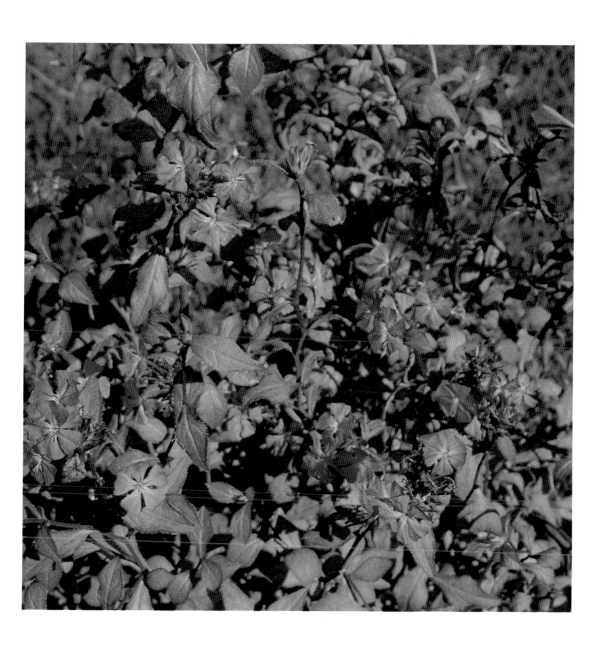

Cerato *Ceratostigma willmottiana*

We come to consider this plant with some uncertainty. It was first brought into this country in 1908 from western China and unlike other introduced species it has not naturalized. If Bach's flowers are to be wild varieties how can we reconcile this contradiction? Bach thought that he might find an English substitute but failed. Although it is now more widely cultivated, in 1930 when Bach first saw this plant in a Cromer garden it was almost unknown. Such exotics were grown by a small band of specialists which presumably included friends of Ellen Willmott, the celebrated Essex gardener who had sponsored the expedition of the plant collector 'Chinese' Wilson. Is it the connection with Tibet that is significant or the five blue petals? It is hard to know where to look for an explanation as to why this flower was chosen as a remedy. Whom can one ask? What would Dr Bach say?

The answer, of course, lies with the plant itself. This is the remedy for those who wish to go forward but are bewildered by uncertainty: they cannot discriminate between right and wrong, between the important and the superficial. As Bach said 'They concentrate too much on the details of life, and miss the main principles: convention and small things count above main issues' *[C.W., 164]*. So it is that uncertainty defines the mental state of the remedy. The plant both poses the question and provides the answer.

The Cerato state of mind seeks an explanation and directive externally when the true source of knowledge and understanding must be internal. This invites us to follow Bach's injunction to listen to the instruction of our soul and not make the mistake of constantly seeking guidance and advice from others who may mislead us. Cerato provides the confidence to trust our own intuition and believe that we can act independently without seeking the support of some external authority. We internalize our attention so that we look to see our own truth.

Locality – Cerato is cultivated in gardens as an ornamental shrub. It is propagated easily by cutting. Specimens can be found in many public gardens such as Kew or Hampton Court (the south garden). It responds to warm, sunny conditions and so will grow best in a sheltered south-facing position. In recent years it has been selected for promotion by some nurseries and has been seen in street gardens in London. However, it is still a specialist's plant.

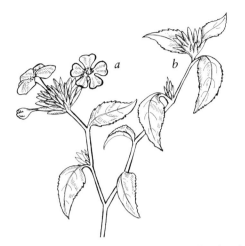 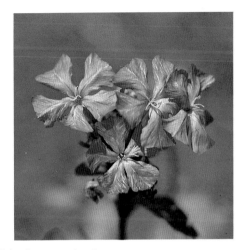

Left: (a) *flower,* (b) *bracts and buds.*   ***Right:*** *detail of the flowering head.*

Identification – Cerato is a small shrub that grows to a height of about 1 m in England. The stems are a reddish brown, the small pointed leaves are covered with short bristling hairs. The flowering heads appear along the stems as a cluster of brown, spiky bracts from which a few flowers appear successively, each lasting only a day. They are bright blue (10-15 cm) with a shade of purple, the small white stamens standing out from the central corolla of the five-petalled flower. It is a small deciduous shrub which is usually pruned back in winter to encourage new growth and so a name-tag may then be the most useful form of indentification.

Flowering Period – from August to early October.

Preparation – Cerato is prepared by the sun method (see p.20). Pick the single flowers within the bract when freshly opened and float them on the bowl of water. To find suitable established plants may not be easy. Specimens can be found in private gardens, but those who wish to meet this plant and its qualities will no doubt obtain one for themselves.

43

CHERRY PLUM

This drives away all the wrong ideas and gives the sufferer mental strength and confidence.

[C.W., 8]

Fear of the mind being over-strained, of reason giving way, of doing fearful and dreaded things, not wished and known wrong, yet there comes the thought and impulse to do them.

[Twelve Healers]

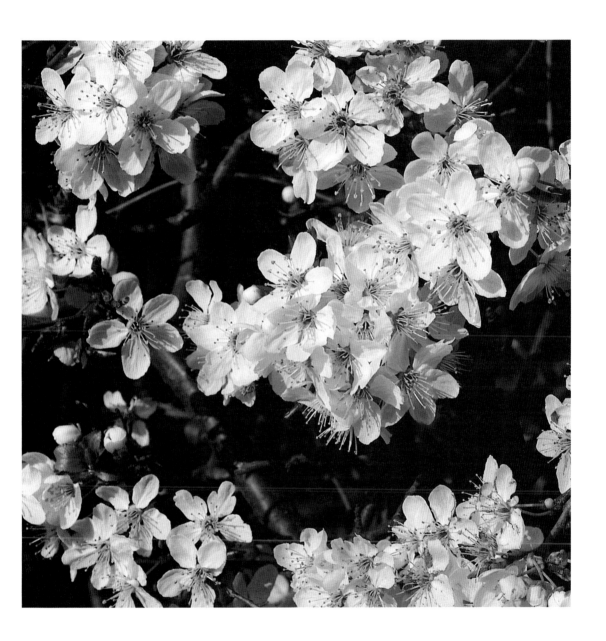

Cherry Plum *Prunus cerasifera*

At the beginning of 1935 Bach embarked upon a new series of remedies, the second nineteen. These, with one exception, were to be prepared by boiling rather than by the sun method. They were discovered in a different manner too in so far as Bach experienced very intensely the negative state of the remedy that was to be found. During March he was successively living with an unknown fear (Aspen), depressed by the enormity of his task (Elm) and terrified that he was going out of his mind (Cherry Plum). This last state with which the season began was accompanied by severe sinus pain and headaches which drove him to distraction. Walking in the lanes around Sotwell he found the white flowers of Cherry Plum growing in the hedge; when he had prepared the essence from them the pain ceased almost with the first drops taken.

It may be unnecessary for us to go to the extreme of being suicidal or in a frenzy of hardly suppressed violence before we appreciate the positive quality of this state: it brings calm, balance and control in any situation. For this reason it forms a part of the rescue remedy combination. When we suffer from the torment of mental stress there is a tendency to lose control, hence the state carries the fear of doing dreadful things. But it is possible, with the help of Cherry Plum, for that desperation to be directed upwards to a harmonious and calm place where the turbulence is quieted, neutralized by the balancing forces of the spirit.

This is a condition in which we need urgently to make contact with our higher self and regain composure. The flowers appear towards the end of winter. Always at that time there are days when clear skies and a bright intense sunshine heralds the hope of spring: Cherry Plum is made on such clear days. With its intensely pure white flowers and buds that barely show the bright green of new leaf it carries a message from the sun of returning life. Like the calm and peace of spring it eases the violence of winter storms. The hedges dressed in white bring forgiveness and reconciliation, expressing the divine command 'Peace! Be still!'

Locality – Cherry Plum was originally brought from the Balkans both for its fruit and as a grafting stock for cultivating more engaging domestic plums. It has not widely naturalized and is noted as rare in some texts. It is more common in the south of England and usually appears in old gardens rather than in scrub woodland (where Sloe will be found). When seen as a hedge it will obviously have been planted there.

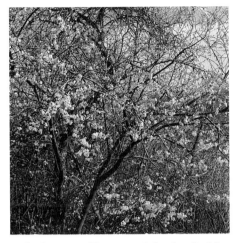 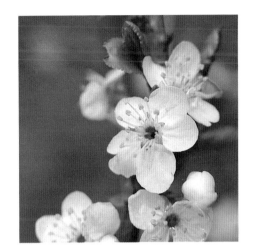

Left: the tree in bloom.　*Right:* detail of flower.

Identification – Cherry Plum is one of a large family of small flowering trees that includes many of the ornamental blossoms of the spring garden. It grows 6-8m high though often it is trimmed for hedging when it suckers easily. The tree grows ragged with a rounded head, and it is generally without thorns. The leaves are oval (2-3cm), toothed and glossy green, appearing after the flowers. The flowers are stalked, pure white, five-petalled (20mm across), with numerous prominent stamens. The fruit, which only sets occasionally, is the colour of ripe tomatoes. This is the first white blossom of the year. It comes out before the Damson or Sloe (*P. spinosa*) with which it might be confused—Sloe has smaller flowers, it is definitely spiked with thorns and has a black (Blackthorn) bark rather than the dull brown of Cherry Plum.

Flowering Period – late February to early April.

Preparation – Cherry Plum is prepared by the boiling method (see p.20). A fine day is particularly important. Twigs of flowers are picked about 15 cm long so as to fit the saucepan.

47

CHESTNUT BUD

AFFIRMATION

We learn slowly, one lesson at a time, but we must if we are to be well and happy, learn the particular lesson given to us by our spiritual self.
[C.W., 157]

INDICATION

For those who do not take full advantage of observation and experience, and who take a longer time than others to learn the lessons of daily life.

Whereas one experience would be enough for some, such people find it necessary to have more, sometimes several, before the lesson is learnt.

Therefore, to their regret, they find themselves having to make the same error on different occasions when once would have been enough, or observation of others could have spared them even that one fault.
[Twelve Healers]

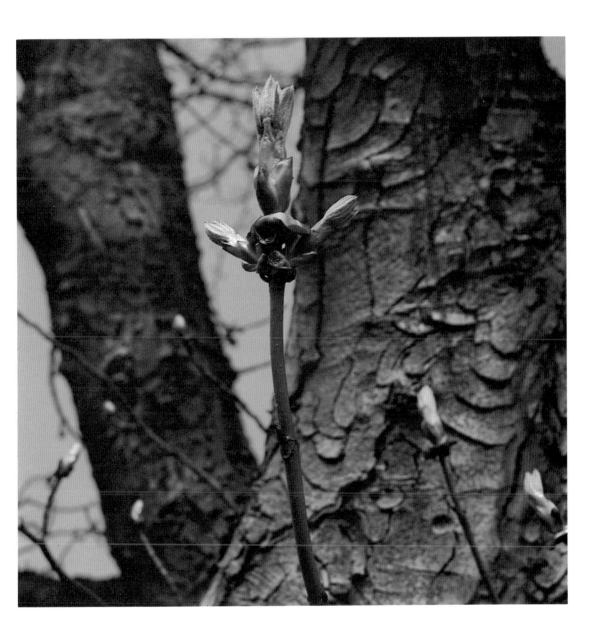

Chestnut Bud   *Aesculus hippocastanum*

If we are to change our lives there must be a moment when a new course is embarked upon. Even the longest journey begins with the decision to go. We base our decisions upon desire and necessity—the carrots and sticks of life. For Bach the matter of listening to our desires was vital: 'our true instincts, desires, likes and dislikes are given us so that we interpret the spiritual commands of our soul...because the soul alone knows what experiences are necessary for that particular personality' *[C.W., 93]*. The sticks of necessity are the proddings of unhappiness and ill health, sure signs that we are not properly attentive to the desire message of our soul. So we are nudged towards life-lessons that are appropriate for us, situations that will help our self-development. There are many ways of trying to avoid the process. Bach characterized some of them in a group of remedy states for *Insufficient Interest in Present Circumstances* and Chestnut Bud, made from the spring buds of the Horse Chestnut, is one of these. It describes a state of mind where we are repeatedly shown something but fail to recognize the pattern and the message that it contains.

'A lack of interest in present circumstances' is another way of saying 'half asleep'. If we are truly alert and awake in the moment then we will observe our circumstances, see what is happening and say 'yes' to the lessons of life. This is a feeling of seeing all things made new and with the freshness of first discovery. It is strong for all of us in spring. Then, each bud that bursts brings a new exploration of existence, although the opening leaves copy perfectly the pattern of their kind. If it were to be the same for us we would be awake in the conscious-ness of the here and now, obervant of the moment and learning the lessons of our kind. As such we would be living strongly into life, powerfully in the present. It is this strength that we can observe in opening buds of the Horse Chestnut. Although they are part of the old tree, set in their form by the development of the last season, they unfold with such force that we can almost see them grow. All bud-burst is potent, but Chestnut Bud is the mightiest. It exemplifies the process of life force active in form pushing out a new future.

Locality – Horse Chestnut trees were brought to Britain from Turkey in the early seventeenth century. They are now found throughout the country, requiring plenty of light and space if they are to develop to full size.

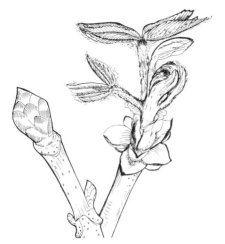 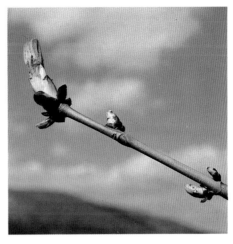

Left: closed buds and emerging leaves.   *Right: the opening bud of Horse Chestnut.*

Identification – Horse Chestnut trees provide the buds for Chestnut Bud. They are well known parkland trees recognizable in winter by the sticky buds and horse-shoe leaf scars. With age the grey-brown bark breaks into rough squares which pull away from the trunk. The opening buds reveal folded emerald green leaves that are coated in creamy down; they are carried on a single, fast growing stem. Leaf buds are in pairs along the twigs while the terminal bud also contains the flower. Chestnut Bud is *not* made from the Red Chestnut, a related variety, that has smaller buds that are smooth and barely sticky, sharply pointed with dull greeny-purple margins. If you recognize Red Chestnut, however, bear it in mind for a later remedy.

Flowering Period – Buds open according to the season, generally early in April.

Preparation – Chestnut Bud is prepared by the boiling method (see p.20). The whole twig is picked (about 15 cm) when the shoot has grown out from the bud but before the leaves have opened. It is a stage of development that needs to be watched for. First the buds swell, then the sticky scales fall back, then the shoot grows out. The resins are part of the remedy; they make a mess of the saucepan which will need to be scoured with a cleaner.

CHICORY

If we but sufficiently develop the quality of losing ourselves in the love and care of those around us, enjoying the glorious adventure of gaining knowledge and helping others, our personal griefs and sufferings rapidly come to an end. It is the great ultimate aim: the losing of our own interests in the service of humanity.
[C.W., 134]

Those who are very mindful of the needs of others; they tend to be over-full of care for children, relatives, friends, always finding something that should be put right. They are continually correcting what they consider wrong, and enjoy doing so. They desire that those for whom they care should be near them.
[Twelve Healers]

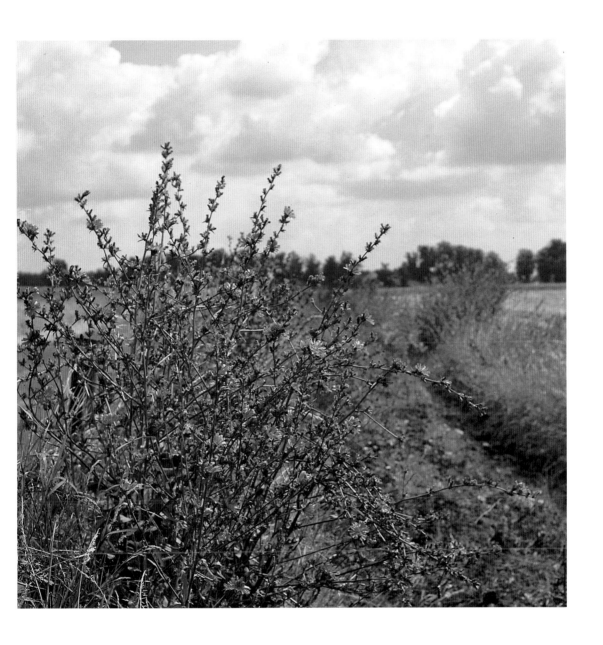

Chicory   *Chicorium intybus*

We may see in this remedy state something of the story of Demeter (or Ceres, or Tullus, or Gaia) the Mother Earth of mythology. In its positive form Chicory is the bountiful expression of the care and love that we can have for all life; the feeling, as Bach put it, that we 'long to open both our arms and bless all around' *[C.W., 104]*. It is this wellspring of love that is essentially found in the mother whether in the family or in the world. It is the image of the receptive, the generous, the forgiving and the devoted: the image of the feminine. Whether in woman or man it involves 'utter forgetfulness of self, the losing of individuality in the Unity' *[C.W., 17]*.

As we all know, however, there are times when love does not flow freely from us. It is not so much that we become angry or jealous but that the active principle of love becomes restrained or congested. Then instead of forgetfulness of self we become obsessed by self, full of self-pity and self-love, self-centred and self-important. The outward impulse of sympathy for others becomes turned inwards and we demand sympathy for ourselves, becoming manipulative and deceitful if we do not receive what we think we deserve.

This condition is expressed in nature by Chicory. The plant commonly grew at the edge of cornfields where Ceres provides for our food. Indeed it has been grown as a fodder crop. The root is used to make a drink and the leaves as a salad vegetable. But it is the flowers that are important in this context. They are a very pure blue which has been spoken of as the blue of devotion, of noble idealism and the blue of spiritual love. Bach thought of it as the blue of Mary, the mother of Jesus. The petals are frail and ragged though the erect styles (which are pale indigo) in the centre of the flower give distinct rays of strength to the stars of colour. It is the strength of the colour that marks Chicory for its unique qualities.

Locality – Chicory grows throughout the south of England especially on calcareous soils. It grows on wasteground, more particularly at the edges of cultivated land, cornfields, or on roadside verges (when they have not been mowed). On more acid soil the flowers are not such an intense blue—they are sensitive as a litmus paper and at times appear pale or even pink after rain, because of the acidity.

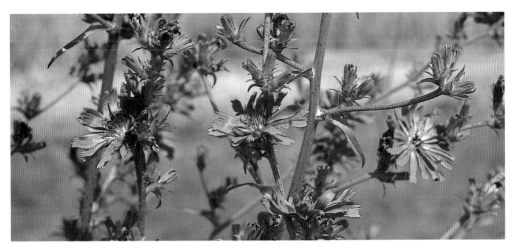
Detail of the flowering stems.

Identification – Chicory grows from a perennial tap root to 1m or more in height forming an open bush with tough branching stems. It is unlike any other plant and is easily recognized by the blue composite flowers (25-40mm). These last only a day, opening at about six o'clock in the morning and closing soon after midday. They are found in the axils of the leaves, a cluster of flower buds which open successively. The leaves and stem are hairy. The lower leaves are large and lobed, somewhat like a large dandelion, the upper leaves are smaller and pointed with the base clasping the stem. Cultivated varieties are similar but with a stronger and more pronounced central stem.

Flowering Period – July to September.

Preparation – Chicory is prepared by the sun method (see p.20). The fully opened flowers are picked from several different plants where they are growing strongly and where the colour is intensely blue. Wild Chicory should be used, taken from a site where it is not contaminated by sprays.

CLEMATIS

AFFIRMATION

The remedy brings stability: and places the patient on a more practical plane; brings them 'down to earth'; and so enables them to fulfil their work in this world.

[C.W., 166]

INDICATION

Those who are dreamy, drowsy, not fully awake, no great interest in life. Quiet people, not really happy in their present circumstances, living more in the future than in the present; living in hopes of happier times, when their ideals may come true. In illness some make little or no effort to get well, and in certain cases may even look forward to death, in the hope of better times; or maybe, meeting again some beloved one whom they have lost.

[Twelve Healers]

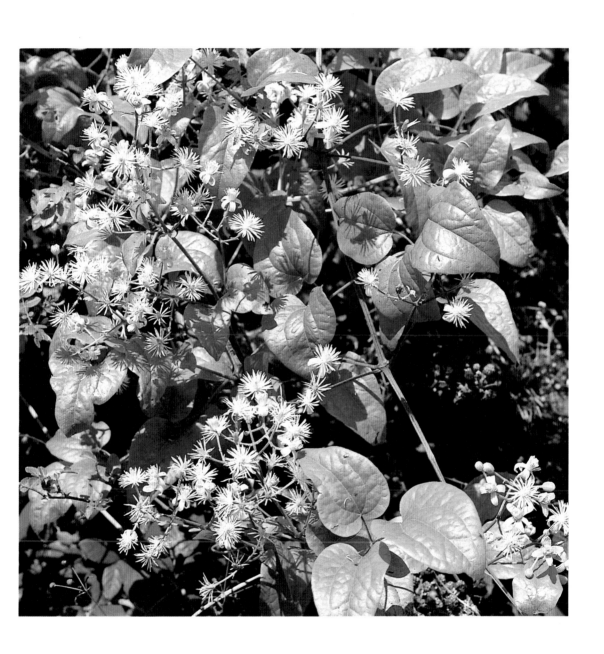

Clematis *Clematis vitalba*

The Latin name *vitalba* means literally white vine: 'white' because of the characteristic silvery white awns of the seeds in early winter and 'vine' because of its habit of climbing over the hedges. Some of the common names are Old Man's Beard (its fluffy appearance) and Travellers' Joy because it grows so prolifically in the lanes and on the roadside; perhaps too for the dried stalks that provide Gypsies' Bacca for the gentlemen of the road! This was one of the first three remedies that Bach identified in 1928; it is for the mentality that is dreamy and not sufficiently awake in the present. It is a creeper that has no means of supporting itself and so it relies upon small trees and shrubs to carry it aloft (think of the firm-rootedness of the Oak for a comparison). The creamy white tufted flowers have no intensity and strength of colour (contrast Gorse or Chicory). As the plant grows it smothers the tree blurring its shape, softening the outline of things, making a cloud of the hedge: clear physical forms become vague and amorphous. In a light breeze the loosely hanging Clematis swings in the wind. Where it lies like a fleecy blanket on the hedge the whole soft mass moves unsteadily. Look at it and you become drawn into its sway; mesmerized by the gentle dream of light and air you too leave the earth and subtly disorientated you are drawn out into another land. The physical world grows remote, faint as smoke and quiet as a fairy dawn. We are in a child's dream.

Mundane reality may be dull by comparison, but this is the life that we must live and we evade human responsibility if we try to escape into fantasy. Bach spoke of this as a polite form of suicide. The soul message is that we must 'come down to earth' and work with life on a more practical plane. If we were supposed to pass this life in the astral worlds then we would have been born there. Yet while Clematis may lead our thoughts into another reality the flower also expresses the purpose of having a strong hold on life. It grows very prolifically and is an extremely successful plant in that it can cover large areas. As it holds on firmly for support it demonstrates our learning 'to hold on when there is nothing in you except the will which says to you—hold on!' *[C.W., 106]*. It grows with the will to be in life.

Locality – Clematis is found throughout southern Britain, though it becomes scarce in the north.

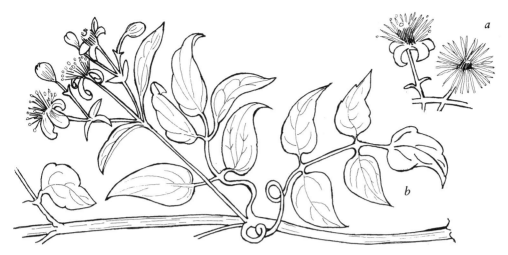

Details: (a) the flower, (b) the pinnate leaf.

Identification – Clematis is a woody perennial growing stems as long as 30 m which hang from trees like jungle vines. The pinnate leaves are pointed (15-20 cm) in opposite pairs on long twisting stalks that serve to entwine branches and provide support since there are no tendrils. Although totally unrelated the White or Black Bryony could be mistaken for Clematis since they also straggle through the hedges, but even a cursory examination will point out the distinction: their leaves are single, the flowers are ranged along a stem and they both form red berries. The creamy white flowers of Clematis are four-petalled (or more properly, sepalled) with numerous very prominent stamens that give a tufted appearance. In autumn the wispy seedheads form the characteristic 'Old Man's Beard'. There are no other wild flower variants of Clematis in Britain—ornamental garden Clematis should not be used.

Flowering Period – July through to September.

Preparation – Clematis is prepared by the sun method (see p.20). Pick the separate flowers by the stalk from several different plants in a place where Clematis is growing strongly. Care should be taken to choose flowers in perfect bloom: this will be apparent by the scent and the pollen on the stamens.

CRAB APPLE

AFFIRMATION

Never for one moment should we become engrossed or over-anxious about them [our bodies], but learn to be as little conscious of their existence as possible, using them as a vehicle of our Soul and mind and as servants to do our will.
[C.W., 151]

INDICATION

This is the remedy of cleansing.

For those who feel as if they had something not quite clean about themselves.

Often it is something of apparently little importance: in others there may be more serious disease which is almost disregarded compared to the one thing on which they concentrate.

In both types they are anxious to be free from the one particular thing which is greatest in their minds and which seems so essential to them that it should be cured.

They become despondent if treatment fails.

Being a cleanser, this remedy purifies wounds if the patient has reason to believe that some poison has entered which must be drawn out.

[Twelve Healers]

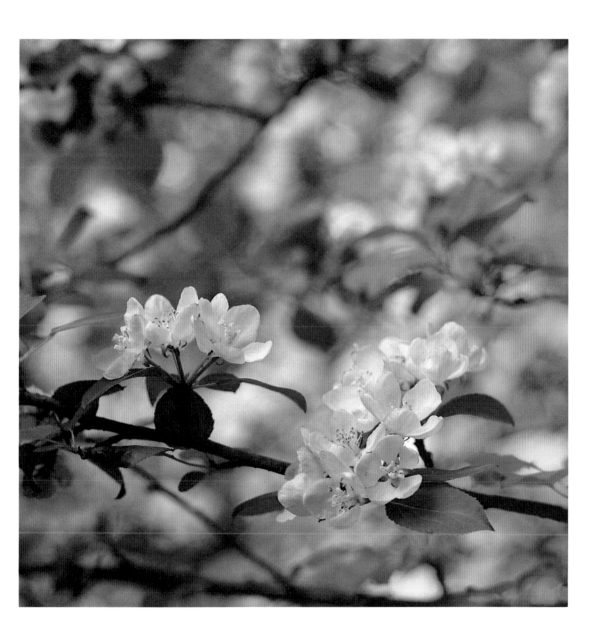

Crab Apple *Malus sylvestris*

Crab Apple is the true wild apple from which domestic varieties were selected and bred. It is not an elegant tree and is unprepossessing to look at. With a wrinkled bark and knotted trunk it is often more bush than tree and can have a scrubby appearance. But as you walk the lanes in May a sweet scent may steal upon you. Look around and you will see in the hedgerow a mass of white blossoms, thronged by bees eager for nectar. There is the Crab Apple, radiant with light, joyfully proclaiming the delight of simple beauty. With all the clear freshness of spring it dispels any petty moods that linger, singing a sweet joy of life, all new and fragrant with brightness like the Morning Star. But this is not a flower of sentimental beauty for it carries a sharp, penetrating clarity—like a shaft of clear white light that acts to purge and cleanse. And while the flowers are sweet the fruit is sharp and bitter: the golden apples of Crab are not what they might seem.

Much of the traditional information concerning apples can be seen to apply to this remedy. It is known that bitter apples in particular carry a healthy weight of minerals, can aid digestion and act to cleanse the system. As a flower remedy Crab Apple is a great stimulant to the life force clearing poisons and bringing renewed activity to the surface of the body. But while, unusually, it is a remedy state that relates to clearing physical problems, its action is predominantly metaphysical. This can be seen in the symbolism associated with apples. Plants represent ideas in a physical form, as the thoughts of the earth; we have myths and legends to tell their story which we call symbolic. So we have myths of apples that give eternal youth, their association with Venus and that beautiful secret they contain: the emblem of immortality, the five-pointed star that can be seen when the apple is cut open. If we remember our immortal self all else falls into place and we can see the small problems of life in a proper perspective.

Locality – Crab Apples are regarded as native to Britain since they probably recolonized the land at the end of the ice age. They are found throughout the country but are scarce in Scotland.

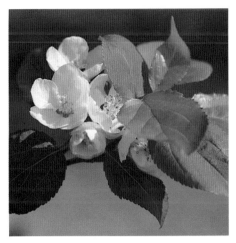 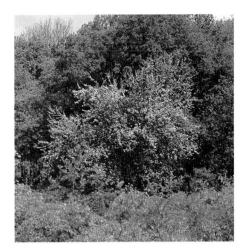

Left: detail of the flowers.   Right: a flowering Crab Apple tree in a hedge.

Identification – Crab Apple is a small tree growing up to 10m. It likes light and space and so will often grow in hedges and clearings where a small group can stand together, self-sown with the help of birds who break up the fruits. Generally it resembles other apples, though the young leaves are only slightly hairy beneath and the young shoots are not covered by woolly down as they are in domestic apples or naturalized cider apples. The dark green leaves (40-50mm) are toothed and often have a partially red stalk, which is more noticeable in autumn when the small golden apples (30-40mm) also make identification easier. The buds are blushed with pink, the flowers white, five-petalled (25mm) and delightfully scented. Like the pear it flowers earlier than domestic apples, though pear blossom has a white bud. There are many ornamental Crab Apples that have been imported for their exotic blossom and fancy fruits and these should be recognized as different. The domestic apple (*M. domestica*) will revert in time to Crab if it seeds into the wild, but the apples are tinged red and not the true golden yellow of the wild Crab Apple.

Flowering Period – May.

Preparation – Crab Apple is prepared by the boiling method (see p.20). Pick the whole cluster of flowers and leaves where they grow at the end of the twigs. Select flowers in perfect bloom from several different trees.

ELM

Life does not demand of us unthinkable sacrifice; it asks us to travel its journey with joy in our heart and to be a blessing to those around, so that if we leave the world just that trifle better for our visit, then have we done our work.
[C.W., 143]

Those who are doing good work, are following the calling of their life and who hope to do something of importance, and this often for the benefit of humanity.

At times there may be periods of depression when they feel that the task they have undertaken is too difficult, and not within the power of a human being.
[Twelve Healers]

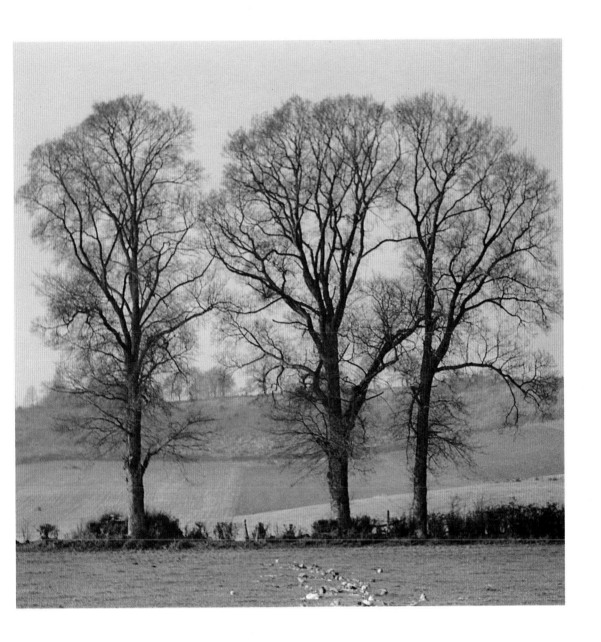

Elm *Ulmus procera*

Whatever can be said of Elm as a remedy it cannot be overlooked that this tree is no longer the characteristic emblem of the English countryside that it once was. The ravages of Dutch Elm Disease have destroyed the majority of the mature trees in the country. The disease, which is endemic in Britain, is a part of the nature of the tree and is itself, in part, an expression of the thought form that the Elm tree represents. Dutch Elm Disease reached epidemic proportions in England in the 1930s at the time that Bach discovered the remedy; it declined after 1936 but returned more virulently in the 1960s. The thought that such handsome and majestic trees could be laid low by a passing fungus seems ironical but the strongest of us can be assailed by weakness. That is the quality of the remedy state—it is for those who are succeeding in life but experience a temporary despondency when they feel they have more responsibility than they can carry and there seems to be a prospect of failure. They do not fail, just as Elm does not become extinct, but the feeling is there nevertheless.

In its positive form the Elm state carries on working despite the difficulties, mindful that the strength is always given for the greatest task. Writing to his colleagues in the month before he died Bach exhorted them: 'Let us forget our limitations, our personalities, our what we think our smallnesses, and let us realize that we have been chosen, picked and special messengers, blessed knights of the highest order...' *[C.W., 31]*. He wanted them to have faith in themselves. Faith is not based upon hopes and beliefs, a comfortable optimism, but the certainty based upon experience. So that Bach was calling for his friends to recognize that what they experienced was proof in itself that they were able to do their work and overcome all difficulties. That had been his experience when, early in 1935, he had doubted that he could fulfil the task of completing the research on his healing herbs and then, seeing the Elm in flower, he had found the strength and conviction to continue and follow it through. The Elm tree has great strength, like the Oak, but it is combined with great sensitivity. We can see this in the fineness of the twigs and the delicate tracery of the branches. But it is the sensitivity that makes it vulnerable.

Locality – Elm once grew throughout Britain but with most of the population lost it is now very localized. A few mature trees can still be found in some northern counties but the disease is killing them rapidly. Young trees are now growing back in most districts. However, it remains to be seen whether they survive.

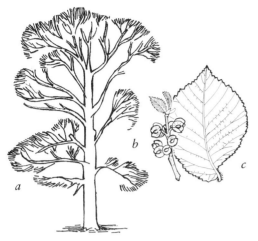
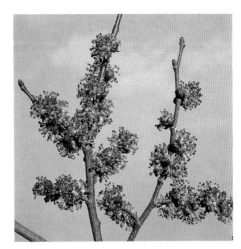

Left: (a) outline of the tree, (b) Elm seeds, (c) the leaf.   Right: detail of the flowers.

Identification – Elm flowers appear before the leaves; small reddish brown clusters smother the branches. The mature tree with its familiar outline is 20-25 m high but it is often seen in hedges. There are many varieties of Elm and care is needed with the identification, especially since the flowers alone do not make a proper distinction. Look out for Wych Elm (*U. glabra*) which is largely unaffected by disease. It is not the one to use, however. The English Elm (*U. procera*) which Bach selected has a similar bark but the tree is taller; it forms suckers, and branches from the column of its trunk while Wych Elm is broader and fan-shaped. Wych Elm has larger seeds and longer, pointed leaves which have a smooth stalk, while the new growth on English Elm is hairy.

Flowering Period – Elm flowers appear in February or March, before the leaves. The trees do not flower profusely every year.

Preparation – Elm is prepared by the boiling method (see p.20). Sections of the twig and flowers are cut so as to fit the saucepan; select from as many different trees as possible. Since the flowers are extremely numerous and are infertile in any case, you will not harm the future prospect of the tree.

GENTIAN

The little Gentian of our hilly pastures will help you to keep your firmness of purpose, and a happier and more hopeful outlook even when the sky is over-cast. It will bring you encouragement at all times, and the understanding that there is no failure when you are doing your utmost, whatever the apparent result.
[C.W., 107]

INDICATION

Those who are easily discouraged. They may be progressing well in illness or in the affairs of their daily life, but any small delay or hindrance to progress causes doubt and soon disheartens them.
[Twelve Healers]

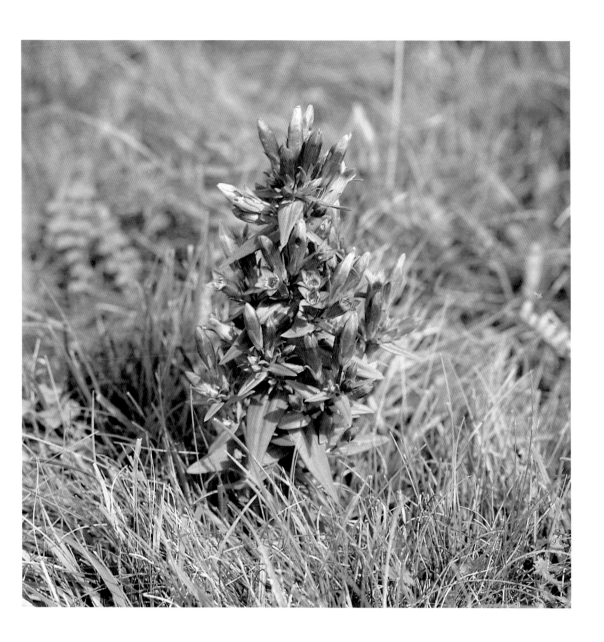

Gentian *Gentiana amarella*

Bach first observed Gentian growing on the chalk hills of Oxfordshire by the path of the Ridgeway. Because it was not yet in flower, he made the remedy elsewhere, on the hills of the Pilgrims Way in Kent. As every type of plant grows in its locality not by chance but as an expression of that place, we can feel some of the qualities of Gentian from the fact that it seeks out hill top grassland in open country. It does not look for the damp lanes in the valley but follows the path that is nearest the sky. From this place we too can look down upon the world and contemplate its ways. Inevitably, we all experience times of difficulty and they can prompt us either to renewed efforts or to discouragement and the expectation of failure. If we can see that we have a tendency to become depressed by our problems it may be that we need to take a bigger view—Bach spoke of it as people's 'desire to go too much their own way, instead of seeing the bigger outlook' *[C.W., 80]*. So the lesson of Gentian is to transform our narrow doubt into understanding.

Of course there are other plants that grow on the Downs as well as Gentian: Centaury and Rock Rose, for instance. So, as well as the matter of location, the colour and structure of the plant can be seen to embody this particular remedy state. It grows alongside the trackways where it is often walked on unwittingly and the seeds trampled into the earth; the young plants lie flat on the grass only growing upwards in the second year. This Gentian, or Autumn Felwort, flowers at the end of the summer, almost too late with its effort one might think. But if the effort is made, it is never too late. As the little towering buds of the Gentian open in the weakening sunshine of September the plant is a small world of intense conviction—few flowers are so physically compact and grow with such solid strength. But if the form of the plant is apparently earthbound, the flower is exotic and the bright purple leads into spiritual realms: it is the colour of inner fulfilment, of majesty, of death and resurrection, the seventh colour of the rainbow. A full understanding of the positive Gentian state leads towards realization. If we go to the place where it grows and sit with the plant we will see that it is so.

Locality – Gentian grows on predominantly calcareous (lime) soils on dry, hill pastures where the grass is short. It will not tolerate farm chemicals and like so many plants, it is, consequently, in retreat.

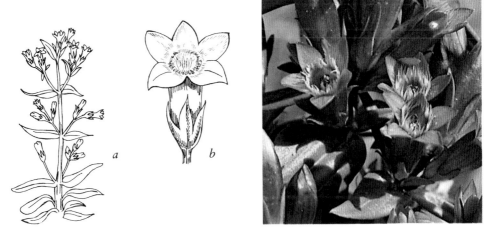

Left: (a) the structure of the plant, (b) detail of a single flower.   Right: detail of the flowers.

Identification – Gentian is a biannual that produces a rosette of leaves in the first year. Then in the second year a short flowering stalk (10-20 cm) with small, purple, trumpet flowers appears. There are five petal-lobes with a white fringe at the throat. The leaves are lanceolate and clasp the stem. Flowers grow from the axil on a short stalk. There are a great many Gentians worldwide but Bach chose this local variety; it flowers only in autumn, it is purple/violet but not blue, nor spotted. The Chiltern Gentian (*G. Germanica*) is similar but with rather larger flowers; like a number of other Felworts it will hybridize.

Flowering Period – from August to early October.

Preparation – Gentian is prepared by the sun method (see p.20). The individual flowers are picked at the top of the stalk and floated on to the bowl of water.

GORSE

Now let us think about those who have been ill for some time, or even a long time. There is again every reason to be hopeful of benefit, either improvement or recovery. Never let anyone give up hope of getting well.

[C.W., 5]

Very great hopelessness, they have given up belief that more can be done for them.

Under persuasion or to please others they may try different treatments, at the same time assuring those around that there is so little hope of relief.

[Twelve Healers]

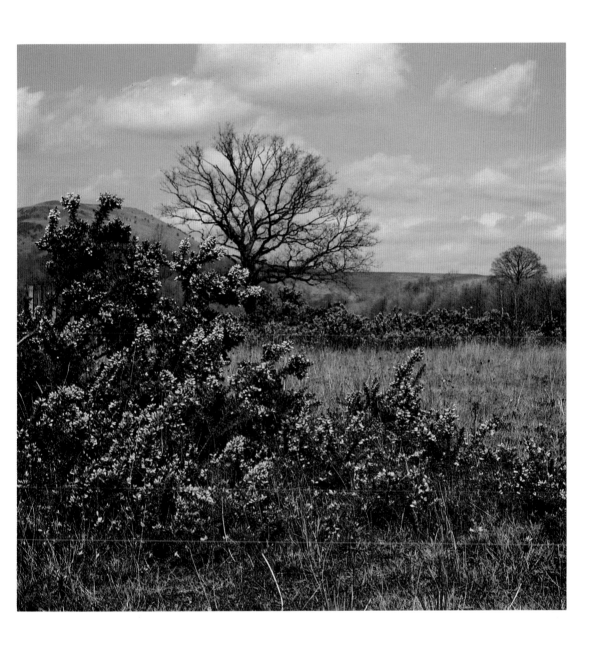

Gorse   *Ulex europaeus*

Each day, each moment, we express in our outlook hope or pessimism; we either affirm life or deny it. There are times when our experience of life has led us to despair, when we lose all hope. And yet we continue to live. We are in a half-life of chronic resignation, for we have lost heart as Bach put it. In such a state no treatment will effect an improvement without a new arousal of the will to live; only when the life force has become reanimated can we hope to improve. Dr Bach recognized that this condition occurred to people who had been ill for a long time, those habituated to their problems, who expected no further improvement, people stuck in a rut. To find a remedy for them he looked for a plant which brought the strength of sunlight ('they look as though they needed more sunshine in their lives to drive away the clouds' *[C. W., 71]*), the strength of purpose to overcome difficulties and the kind of protection that would give the courage to fight. This plant was Gorse.

Gorse carries the strength of the sun in its golden yellow flowers. When it is in full bloom early in the spring it has a charge of brilliant intensity that awakens the land to new hope and new life. Many other spring flowers echo this yellow. They bring in the yellow light: combined with the blue winter darkness it leads to the fresh green of summer. But Gorse has been in flower a little throughout the winter, withstanding the cold and snow: even at the solstice it was a signal of new life. Hope may grow faint but it never dies. This resilience is given protection: to prevent animals eating the flowers Gorse has mighty spines which defend it and those who shelter in its undergrowth. It is a very lion of golden strength, certainty and confidence.

Locality – Gorse can be found throughout Britain. It grows on most soils but will avoid chalk and lime, preferring the slight acidity of moorlands and dry sandy commons. In summer the ripe seeds explode and so a thick clump of Gorse will slowly spread and dominate an area.

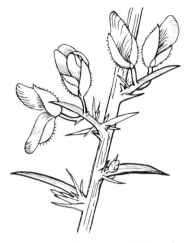 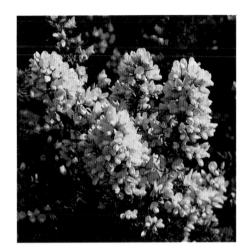

Left: *the leaves and flowers.*   **Right:** *a flowering branch.*

Identification – There are only three types of Gorse and while there are differences in size and colour they are similar in their appearance...a very prickly evergreen bush! *U. europaeus*, which Bach chose, is the largest Gorse, up to 2m high with many branches which are covered in strong sharp spines (10-20mm). The smaller Gorses (*U. minor* and *U. gallii*) both flower later in the year, often making a rich display with the Heather in September. Their flowers are not so golden being rather a bright pale yellow like the Broom. Broom is a related shrub which has no spines and small rounded leaves.

Flowering Period – Although it is true that Gorse may flower throughout the year it is abundant in spring and early summer, from late March to early June.

Preparation – Gorse is prepared by the sun method (see p.20). Choose a place where Gorse is prolific and select from bushes throughout the clump. The flowers are picked by the short stalk and floated on to the water. Bach said that the blooms should be taken just before Gorse reaches its full glory, a little before it gives out scent, probably in mid April.

HEATHER

We must steadfastly practise peace, imagining our minds as a lake ever to be kept calm, without waves, or even ripples, to disturb its tranquillity and gradually develop this state of peace until no event of life, no circumstance, no other personality is able under any circumstances to ruffle the surface of that lake....
[C.W., 152]

INDICATION

Those who are always seeking the companionship of anyone who may be available, as they find it necessary to discuss their own affairs with others, no matter whom it may be. They are unhappy if they have to be alone for any length of time.
[Twelve Healers]

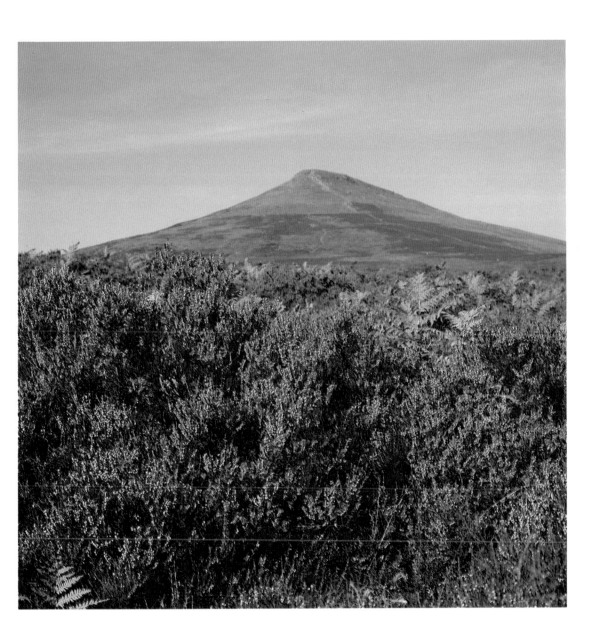

Heather *Calluna vulgaris*

Most of us live in towns and cities. We exist in tight confinement, pressed in upon ourselves by a crowded urban life. And, for the most part, all of us become a little self-obsessed. We live our lives rooting among our own concerns, fussing over our problems, keeping on about our small lives as if nothing else mattered. Natural enough apparently! Yet, as we become driven in upon ourselves we can become lonely. We fill our minds with thought and desperately seek others to share those thoughts with; or we look outside to find people whose problems can help to fill our emptiness. This state of affairs is not natural. As Bach describes it this is a chronic state of difficulty which overlies and disguises our true personality. We have only to imagine the tranquillity of a clear night sky, the quiet depth of a peaceful lake or the calm meditative silence of the mountains to understand why. Pressed in between the buildings we easily forget about the places where the wilderness remains. We end up fearing them as we fear the wilderness of the soul.

The plant that grows in the wilderness of Britain is Heather. Its pink and purple flowers cover the mountains at the end of summer like a gentle fire drawing down the blessing that satisfies our inner longing and loneliness. Bach wrote that this remedy calms fears and soothes the anxieties of those who are overconcerned by petty details. Heather tolerates the exposure of moorland, withstands the bleakness of poor, thin soils and thrives where few other plants can. It does so by becoming self-reliant; growing in spreading clumps the tiny flowers are a mass of busy chatter like a miniature forest. In a lifetime of twenty to thirty years the low bush will smother all other plants and poison the soil with acidity. So it carries both the positive and negative aspects of the emotional state: it can survive the loneliness and yet it prevents other plants from living near to it. But the thought that it embodies brings integration so that we can find in ourselves what we would seek from others, and can allow to others what will truly fulfil ourselves.

Locality – Heathers grow on many infertile soils throughout Britain. They like acidity and tolerate both wet, boggy ground and dry, sandy heaths. They are most obviously found in mountains and moorland. Bach mentions the mountains of Scotland and Wales although Devon or Yorkshire would do equally well. The photograph overpage shows the Suger Loaf, in Gwent.

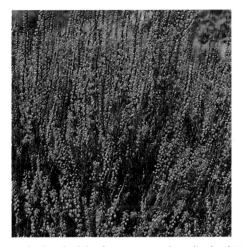 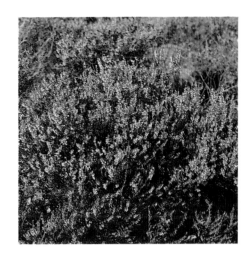

Left: *detail of the flowers.*   ***Right:*** *a bush of Heather.*

Identification – There is only one *Calluna vulgaris* although a few other plants (the *Ericas*) grow in the same situation and need to be recognized as different. *Calluna vulgaris* is a woody evergreen with very small, narrow leaves in dense opposite rows along the stems while *Ericas* have leaves in whorls, grouped up the stem. The pink and purple flowers are small and four-petalled while the *Ericas* have red or pale pink flowers shaped like a flask or bell. Reference to a *Flora* will quickly point out the differences and clarify any confusion over the local names that are given to Heather.

Flowering Period – August and September, at the end of the summer.

Preparation – Heather is prepared by the sun method (see p.20).With this remedy only, Bach said originally that it could be prepared after midday. The flowering stems are taken in full bloom, without too many buds and without any dying flowers or those that have gone to seed. The sprigs are floated on to the water bowl. Collect from many different plants from around the mass of the Heather patch. Garden varieties should not be used.

HOLLY

AFFIRMATION

The ultimate conquest of all will be through love and gentleness, and when we have sufficiently developed these two qualities nothing will be able to assail us, since we shall ever have compassion and not offer resistance.

[C.W., 135]

INDICATION

For those who are sometimes attacked by thoughts of such kind as jealousy, envy, revenge, suspicion.

For the different forms of vexation.

Within themselves they may suffer much, often when there is no real cause for their unhappiness.

[Twelve Healers]

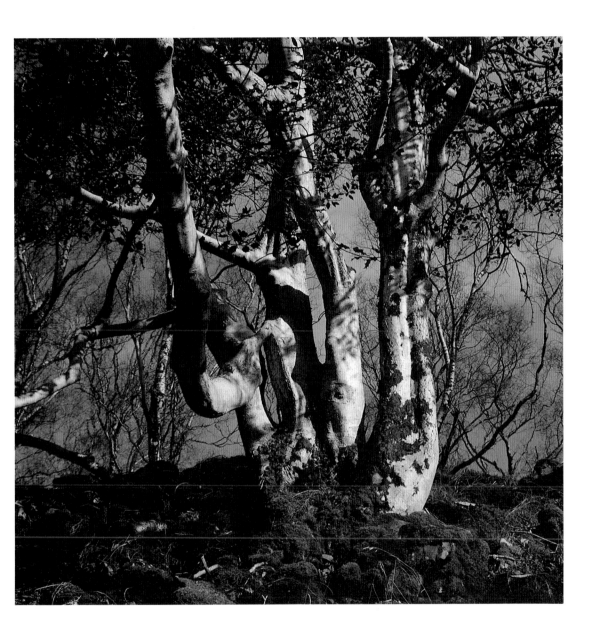

Holly *Ilex aquifolium*

The Thirty-Eight Remedy States are grouped under seven headings—that for Holly is *Oversensitivity to Ideas & Influences*. Like Walnut, the Holly tree offers protection, protection from negative influences that can attack, or rather, possess us. While Walnut protects from outside influences, Holly protects us from influences that have become internal. We do not like being jealous or angry; we all prefer happiness to rage. But at times we become helplessly overwhelmed by negativity. It comes into us as a malevolent thought pattern (the image of a demon has been used by storytellers) that takes us over, often taking up permanent residence within us. When this occurs we become unrecognizable, our natural face is contorted by antipathy, we set ourselves against everything even when there is no real cause. Envy, hatred, vexation or jealousy can attack any one of us. If we are alert we will resist the attack by a conscious movement of the heart which counters with love. But should we be too open to such negative influences we will become prisoners in our own mind.

There is a strong tradition that associates Holly with the power to ward off evil. Whether it is in the Roman rites of Saturnalia, through the Druids or the Christian Church matters little. There are few other native evergreen broadleafed trees and Holly is special for that alone, having a reputation for immortality since it keeps its leaves throughout the year. It grows slowly but with great purpose and strength, forming impenetrable hedges. The tough waxy leaves show its vitality. In a practical sense the spines that are so prominent on the lower leaves are there to prevent animals from eating them, but this physical protection is emblematic of a more subtle protection that the tree embodies. Bach spoke of the remedies found in 1935 (the second nineteen) as 'more spiritualized', more able to 'develop that inner great self' that has the power to overcome our life difficulties. Thus Holly acts to reunite us with our own self, to drive out the negativity and flood us with the healing vibrations of love. Its action is protective but it is also transforming. We can see this more in the sweetness of the flower than in the sharpness of the leaves. When the buds open in May the bees throng the tree for nectar, drawn by the delicate scent. Sweet-scented flowers always stir the heart.

Locality – Holly grows throughout Britain but it is rather less common in the eastern counties. It grows in thickets and woodland, being seeded by birds.

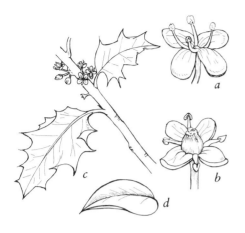
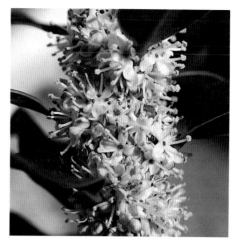

Left: flowers (a) male, (b) female; (c) leaf with spines, (d) smooth leaf.   Right: a flowering branch.

Identification – Holly is a common evergreen tree or bush growing up to 20 m with a smooth, grey bark. It is best recognized by the spiked leaves. These are generally less spiny higher up the tree and in old Hollies spines may be quite absent. The flowers are small, white and four-petalled, tinged with pink and very fragrant. Trees are generally either wholly male or female (which is the reason why some trees do not bear fruit). Male flowers are slightly larger with prominent stamens, the female have rudimentary stamens and a large pistil that will be the berry. There are many ornamental Hollies which should not be used.

Flowering Period – May to June.

Preparation – Holly is prepared by the boiling method (see p.20). The flowering twigs are picked so as to fit the saucepan. Male or female flowers can be used but select from several different trees. The leaves are bulky and get in the way somewhat but a few should be included.

HONEYSUCKLE

AFFIRMATION

Finally, let us not fear to plunge into life; we are here to gain experience and knowledge, and we shall learn but little unless we face realities and seek to our utmost.

[C.W., 138]

INDICATION

Those who live much in the past, perhaps in a time of great happiness, or memories of a lost friend, or ambitions which have not come true. They do not expect further happiness such as they have had.

[Twelve Healers]

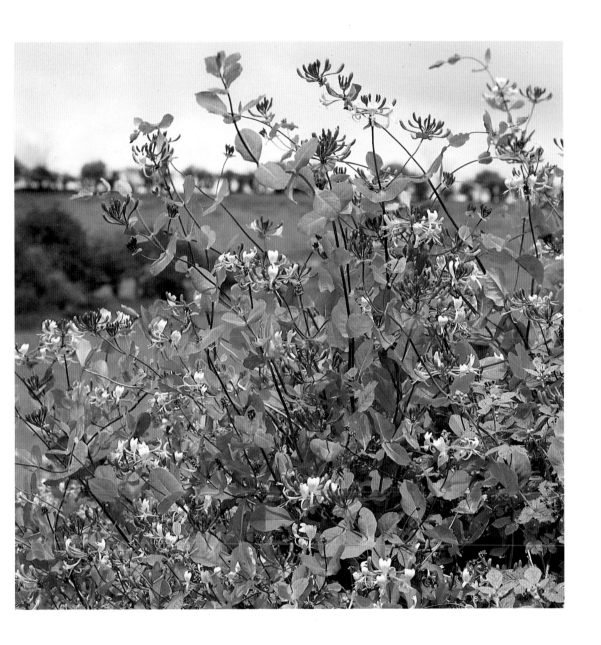

Honeysuckle *Lonicera caprifolium*

Janus, one of the oldest Latin Gods, was thought to have two faces: one looked back at the past, one looked towards the future. We gave the name January to the first month of the year because Janus supervised the beginning of new events and the entry into places. All of these attributes are associated strongly with the Honeysuckle state. As it is a member of the plant family *Caprifoliaceae* we can see a link to Capricorn and so to January—not because goats like the plant but because Honeysuckle begins to open new leaves in January. It often grows as an ornamental arch over a cottage path where Janus was invoked as the god of gateways. Most of all Honeysuckle is the remedy for those who live too much in the past, who are more active in their memories than in the prospect of a new opportunity. While it is essential that we learn from the past (Chestnut Bud speaks of that) this condition carries a longing to be back in the past, in a situation that appears to have been more attractive than our current circumstances. In this Honeysuckle state we live in our thoughts and give of our life force to the images that are held in our astral bodies, like dreams. Consequently we live less and less in life, more and more in those things that are dead and gone.

When recognizing Honeysuckle as an expression of this mentality Bach chose one particular type of plant: the red one that is not the native English flower. The yellow flower has the sweet softness and romanticism of a 'luscious woodbine' bower in *A Midsummer Night's Dream*, a fairy enchanter. But the power of the red forcibly brings us out of that condition and thrusts us into the present, so we can look with the other face of Janus, towards the future. The bursting vitality of the blood red corolla displays a pure lining of white, curling open to reveal the delicate filaments of the stamens. Tiny trumpets, they declare the now.

Locality – Red Honeysuckles are either wild hybrids or garden escapes. They were introduced from Holland where this bright red variety grows. Because it is the redness allied to the pattern of growth that gives its quality, a garden plant will embody the nature of this remedy state. It often grows strongly in an old cottage garden. Wild plants, though uncommon, can be found in woodlands and hedges in south east England.

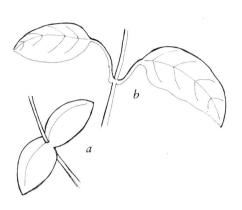
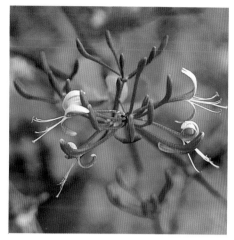

Left: (a) perfoliate leaf, (b) stemmed leaf of common Honeysuckle.   Right: flowering head.

Identification – Honeysuckle is a trailing perennial climber that covers hedges and small trees, growing up to 6 m in length. The leaves are rounded in opposite pairs, the flowers bud at the end of the stem in a cluster of lengthening red tubes that split open to reveal the stamens and style. The inside of the tube is white but it turns yellow when the flower has been pollinated. The distinction that is made between *L. caprifolium* and *L. periclymenum* can be seen in the leaves. *L. caprifolium*, which Bach chose, has perfoliate leaves (only on the upper stems), that is they clasp around the stem without a stalk.   *L. periclymenum* also has a pink variety so the leaves should be examined carefully. Fly Honeysuckle (*L. xylosteum*) has yellowish flowers in pairs, it is smaller and has pointed leaves.

Flowering period – June to August.

Preparation – Honeysuckle is prepared by the boiling method (see p.20). The flowering heads are picked with a few leaves. Select those flowers that are predominantly red and white without too many of the dying yellowed petals.

HORNBEAM

Thus every moment of our work and play will bring with it a zeal for learning, a desire to experience real things, real adventures and deeds worth-while....
[C.W., 149]

INDICATION

For those who feel that they have not sufficient strength, mentally or physically, to carry the burden of life placed upon them; the affairs of every day seem too much for them to accomplish, though they generally succeed in fulfilling their task.

For those who believe that some part, of mind or body, needs to be strengthened before they can easily fulfil their work.

[Twelve Healers]

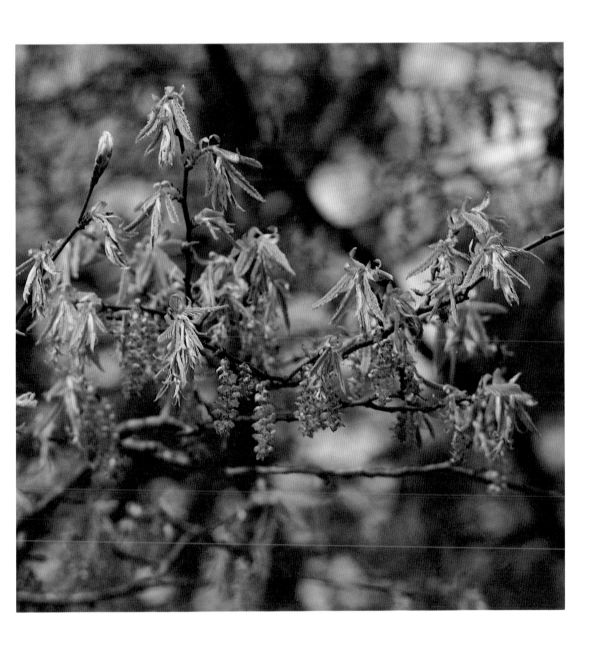

Hornbeam *Carpinus betula*

Hornbeam is a strong tree. As a remedy it strengthens us when we feel that we are unable to get going, unable to carry the weight of our daily lives. While Olive is for real exhaustion Hornbeam is for the feeling of being tired. There is little in its symbolism to indicate that this is so. Although it is a handsome tree, of medium size, attractive throughout the year with the pagoda-shaped bracts that surround the female flowers, it is otherwise unremarkable. In its practical applications, however, we can see the strength of the Hornbeam. The wood is exceptionally hard and smooth, white like horn or bone, it is very strong and able to withstand much wear. It now functions as little more than an ornamental tree but Hornbeam was once used extensively: for mallets, skittles, in cartwheels, for cog wheels in mills, as yokes for oxen pulling a plough, for the delicate moving parts of a piano, and as a hard and unyielding block for butchers to chop meat upon. These were the strange and varied purposes for which this timber was especially useful; collectively they denote a character of strength, utility and good purpose. That is the nature of the positive Hornbeam state. It has staying power, true determination to work and get on with what needs to be done.

It is an adaptable tree and has allowed itself to be trained into arches and leafy bowers: the Hornbeam Walk at Hampton Court is an example. This is a curiosity worth experiencing since it concentrates the Hornbeam pattern into a tunnel that you can walk through. The dense foliage provides a cool shade, the dynamic of the tree provides a boosting vitality. It is a hardy tree, indifferent to the vagaries of the soil, tolerant of harsh winds and able to withstand the wood cutters—at one time the Hornbeams of Epping Forest were coppiced to provide fuel for local people who were granted a licence by Queen Elizabeth I. The timber makes very good logs.

Locality – Hornbeam grows wild only in south east England; elsewhere in Britain it is planted. It is found throughout the Home Counties (around London) especially in Hertfordshire and in Epping and Hainault Forests. Bach found it growing in the Thames Valley.

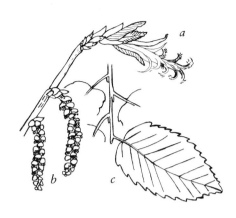 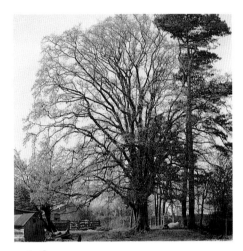

Left: *flowers (a) female, (b) male; (c) leaf.*   **Right:** *the tree in flower.*

Identification – Hornbeam grows up to about 20m and in some respects might be mistaken for Beech. The leaves are similar but distinctly toothed, somewhat like a smooth Elm leaf. The smooth bark of the trunk has characteristic grey streaks unlike any other tree. The flowers are often very numerous and showy; male and females appear on the same tree although one or other may predominate. The males are yellow catkins, the females are smaller with unusual curving bracts. These grow to form a three-pointed wing for flight to carry the seed away from the tree.

Flowering Period – April and May. It does not flower strongly every year.

Preparation – Hornbeam is prepared by the boiling method (see p.20). Pick twigs with both male and female flowers, gathering them from as many different trees as possible.

IMPATIENS

AFFIRMATION

You are striving for exquisite gentleness and forgiveness, and that beautiful mauve flower, Impatiens, which grows along the sides of some of the Welsh streams, will, with its blessing, help you along the road.

[C.W., 108]

INDICATION

Those who are quick in thought and action and who wish all things to be done without hesitation or delay. When ill they are anxious for a hasty recovery.

They find it very difficult to be patient with people who are slow, as they consider it wrong and a waste of time, and they will endeavour to make such people quicker in all ways.

They often prefer to work and think alone, so that they can do everything at their own speed.

[Twelve Healers]

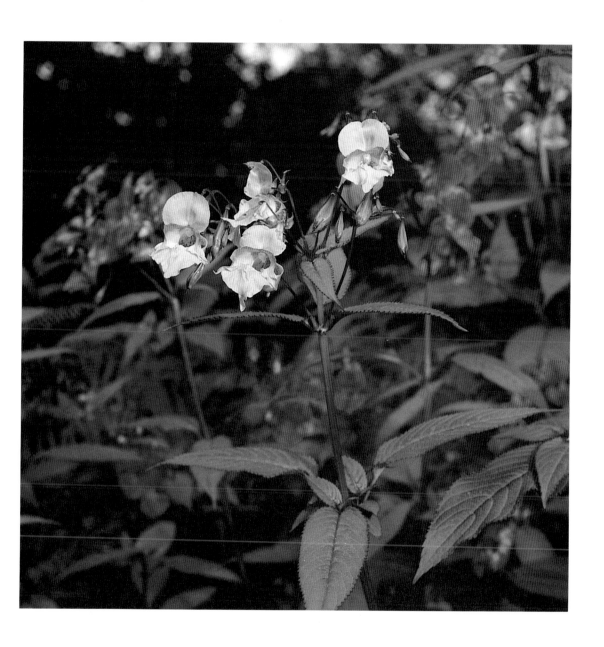

Impatiens   *Impatiens glandulifera*

Impatiens was probably the first flower remedy that Dr Bach identified. Visiting Wales in 1928 he saw this Himalayan Balsam growing on a riverbank along with Mimulus (see p.98). Significantly, neither plant is a British native. *Impatiens glandulifera* was found in Kashmir in the 1830s and brought back to England. It escaped and has been so successful as a colonist that it has now become common throughout the country. Apparently it is still on the increase. It is for the emotional state of irritation, for tension and pain. The pattern of growth that the plant displays can be used to explain why this is so and to illustrate other aspects of the remedy state.

Bach first saw Impatiens in late September when the pods were ripe; no doubt he observed how they exploded and scattered the seeds like little bullets. The sides of the pod are elastic and they curl back like tiny writhing snakes—to experience this just take hold of one of the fat pointed pods and it will give a perfect demonstration of the explosive irritation of Impatiens! The seeds need the cold of winter before germination but they are quick off the mark in spring and soon outgrow other plants. That is why Impatiens grows so densely and forms such a bank of flowers. Bach observed that the Impatiens person likes to work alone, at speed and without interference, just like the plant.

The plants are tall, branched and leafy with brittle fleshy stems growing up to 2m in a few months. The flowers are amazingly delicate for such a powerful plant and they hang from a fine stalk, poised and balanced, with an open mouth inviting insects. Constantly active Impatiens carries buds, flowers and seeds simultaneously through the late summer. Most of the flowers are a hot mauve colour, a mottled deep red. But Bach specified that only the pale mauve flowers were to be used in preparing a remedy. The reason for this is that they are cooler and more delicate, carrying the essence of the sweet, gentle, relaxed tenderness that is characteristic of the positive state of Impatiens.

Locality – Impatiens is found throughout Britain. It grows along the banks of streams and rivers, the seeds travelling in the water. It will grow in full light or shade and accepts varying soils, unless markedly acid. It prefers damp ground.

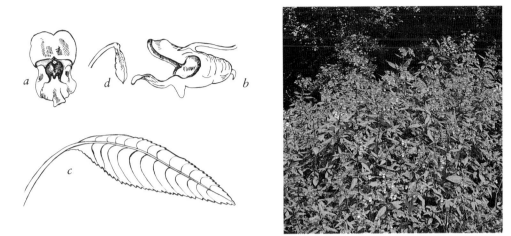

Left: details of the flower (a) front, (b) side view, (c) leaf, (d) seedpod.   *Right:* a bank of Impatiens.

Identification – *Impatiens glandulifera* (also known as *I. roylei*) is the only plant of its kind although there are two or three other Balsams that are related. It grows tallest and strongest of the family, the others have yellow or orange flowers. It is a fast growing annual, the leaves are large and pointed with a toothed edge, dark green and like the stem they are lined in purple. The flowerheads are carried on stems that spring from the base of the leaves. The five petals are fused to form a hood or helmet (it is sometimes called Policeman's Helmet). This Impatiens is not the same as the popular houseplant called 'Busy Lizzie'.

Flowering period – July to September, or up until the frost.

Preparation – Impatiens is prepared by the sun method (see p.20). Only the pale mauve flowers are used; pick them by the slender stalks and float them on to the water. Choose a place where the flowers grow really strongly and select from several different plants.

LARCH

AFFIRMATION

We chose the earthly occupation, and the external circumstances that will give us the best oppportunities of testing us to the full: we come with the full realization of our particular work: we come with the unthinkable privilege of knowing that all our battles are won before they are fought, that victory is certain before ever the test arrives, because we know that we are children of the Creator, and as such are Divine, unconquerable and invincible.

[C.W., 91]

INDICATION

For those who do not consider themselves as good or capable as those around them, who expect failure, who feel they will never be a success, and so do not venture or make a strong enough attempt to succeed.

[Twelve Healers]

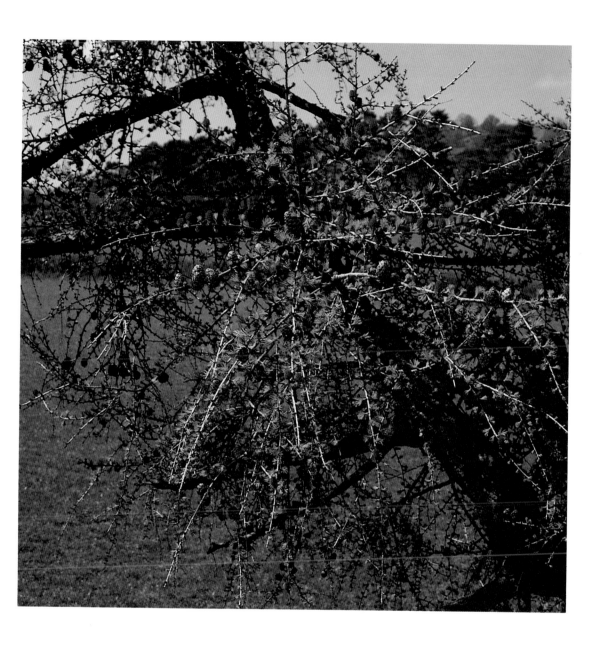

Larch   *Larix decidua*

Larch trees have an air of despondency, especially in autumn when they appear to be dying—unlike other conifers they shed their leaves. The branches droop in a languid manner and seem reluctant to straighten up with the determination needed for a strong growth. Such is the Larch state. Although we may be perfectly capable we allow a lack of confidence to direct us; expecting failure we do not make the effort to succeed. There is no doubt that all of us have been acquainted with such a state of mind. But we may wonder why the Larch tree offers the antidote. Some people may feel that although Bach recognized it, they would lack the confidence to approach the question for themselves...! If we can learn the lesson of the Larch we can see the pattern that lies within all the remedies—it is not beyond any of us, we just need the confidence to try and see it.

The Larch tree grows very quickly and strongly; like other conifers it is straight and tall although the slender top of the trunk curves gracefully, unable to hold itself erect. Its appearance is strangely vague. The fineness of the leaves, the sweeping gesture of the branches, the sketchy tracery and unfocused outline make it tentative, uncertain. The leaf shoots are amongst the first in spring and the little tufts of soft needles slowly colour up the drooping twigs; Larch creeps diffidently into green. The flowers are modest, yet looked at closely they are exquisitely structured with a delicacy and strength that characterizes the positive Larch state. Here is a being that looks to be one thing yet is in fact quite different. Larch was brought to England in the early seventeenth century from the mountain regions of central Europe. There it was adapted to a brief summer growing period and harsh winters. It is a native of the tundra where the permafrost of winter freezes the ground so that no water at all can be taken up into the trees; they must shed their leaves to survive. While Larch appears to be delicate it is actually resilient and able to withstand extremes. Like the Larch people it is a good deal more capable than it appears.

Locality – Larch is not a native of Britain but has been widely planted, especially as a plantation tree for commercial purposes. It prefers well-drained ground and avoids extremes of acid or alkaline soils.

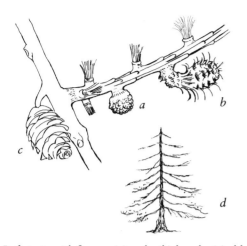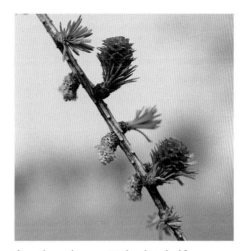

Left: twig with flowers (a) male, (b) female; (c) old cone, (d) outline of tree. **Right:** *detail of flowers.*

Identification – Larch is a characteristic tree of 30 m or more. It has a straight, tapering trunk with rough bark, the branches grow out at right angles from the trunk and droop in a curve, the tips pointing upwards. Leaves are in tufts of green needles. Flowers of both sexes are found on the same tree: females are red, males yellow. Egg-shaped cones remain on the branches from previous years. Many varieties of Larch can be found. The Japanese Larch *L. kaempferi* has only yellow flowers while the hybrid Dunkeld Larch *L.* × *eurolepis*, which was developed to resist disease is more slender with twigs that are grey rather than straw yellow. It is a variable form with flowers ranging from purple to cream tinged in red. Dahurian, American and Western Larch are also grown. But the Common Larch *L. decidua*, which Bach chose, is still the most usual form of mature tree outside of forestry areas.

Flowering Period – late March and April.

Preparation – Larch is prepared by the boiling method (see p.20). Twigs are picked from as many different trees as possible. Both male and female flowers are collected, with young leaves, on twigs about 15 cm long, so as to fit the saucepan.

99

MIMULUS

Fear in reality holds no place in the natural human kingdom, since the Divinity within us, which is ourself, is unconquerable and immortal, and if we could but realize it we, as Children of God, have nothing of which to be afraid.
[C.W.,149]

Fear of worldly things, illness, pain, accidents, poverty, of dark, of being alone, of misfortune. The fears of everyday life. These people quietly and secretly bear their dread, they do not speak freely of it to others.
[Twelve Healers]

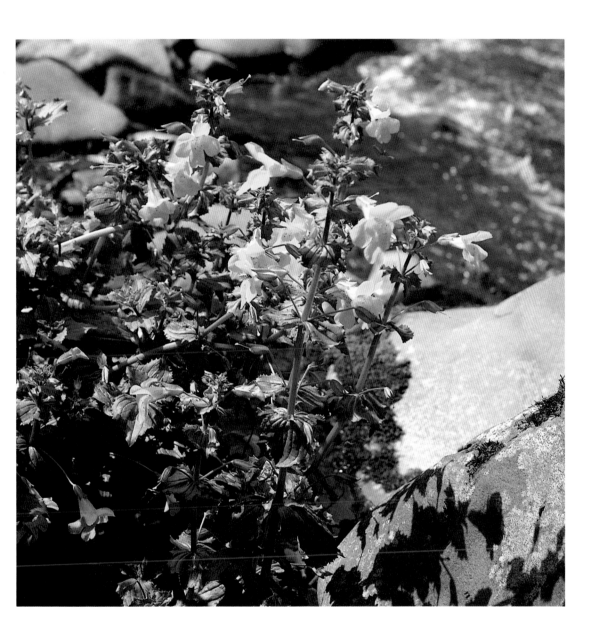

Mimulus   *Mimulus guttatus*

Mimulus or Monkey Flower was one of the first three remedies found by Dr Bach when he was searching for plants along the River Usk in 1928. It was introduced into Britain from North America early in the nineteenth century. The first report of its having escaped to the wild was in 1824 when it was found growing near the Welsh border town of Abergavenny. It is the remedy for nervousness and fear, fears of a known origin. Every plant is an expression of the place where it grows and, at the same time, its particular qualities encourage it to seek out the habitat where its nature will find a full expression. Thus, while some flowers grow in the fields and others in woodland, Mimulus is found clinging to the stones on a riverbank, precariously hanging over the water where it is constantly splashed and washed by the stream. Once established, the plant roots down into the bed of gravel and, knowing no fear, it withstands the dangers of growing half in the water.

Fear is a state of mind that will not let go and trust to life. Bach spoke of fear as being more prevalent in our materialistic age because we place importance on earthly possessions, whether the body itself or external riches. Everything on earth is transient so we tend to live in fear of what we may lose or fail to gain. Mimulus, however, sets an example of how we may live happily amongst dangers and find freedom through the acceptance of our situation, being vulnerable, yet setting love of life above our fear. Mimulus takes a great risk. Its thousands of tiny seeds fall into the water and are washed away. Yet some lodge along the bank and in the stones a new plant grows up. Like the grass that grows on the weir we can take life easy and live it as it comes. By the crystal stream, with the sound of water constantly singing its joyful melody of life, there is no fear. This joy is expressed by the water in the bright green leaves of the Mimulus and its delicate bright yellow flowers: confident, happy, with a smile of sympathy and peace.

Locality – Mimulus grows on wet ground and watercourses throughout Britain. But it is becoming more local as it will not tolerate the chemical pollution that washes into most streams and rivers from farmland. Where Bach found Mimulus 'growing to perfection' along the River Usk it is now little in evidence. He spoke of 'crystal streams where the water is clear'—they are now a rarity in lowland Britain.

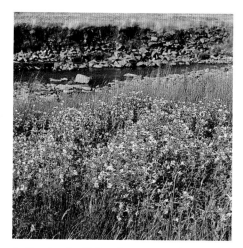
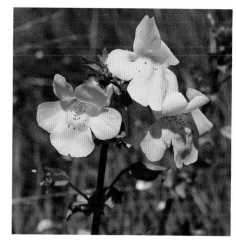

Left: a bank of Mimulus growing by a Welsh stream. **Right:** *detail of the flower.*

Identification – Mimulus grows with the fleshy green stems of a water plant to a height of about 50 cm, the leaves are opposite and clasp the stem. Flowers are five-petalled but they fuse to form an open mouth, about 25-30 mm; they are bright yellow with a few red spots on the lower lip. Bach originally nominated the yellow flower as *M. luteus* but it was later identified as *M. guttatus*.* The Blood-drop Emlets, *M. luteus*, is a similar flower from Chile, being smaller with a distinctly red-spotted flower. The two species hybridize freely with the red *M. luteus* appearing to dominate the yellow *M. guttatus*. In adjacent valleys the two may grow separately but when they meet downstream the yellow flowers will be darker with more red spots. Plant breeders too are creating hybrids and as these in turn escape and cross pollinate they alter the natural plant form. The yellow *M. guttatus* is the one to use.

Flowering Period – from June through to August.

Preparation – Mimulus is prepared by the sun method (see p.20). Find a place where the wild flowers are growing strongly by a bright stream and select from several different plants. Pick the flowers by their stalks and float them on to the surface of the water bowl.

---

* The Latin name was changed in the 1952 edition of *The Twelve Healers & Other Remedies* in accordance with changes in the International Rules of Botanical Nomenclature.

MUSTARD

In all things cheerfulness should be encouraged, and we should refuse to be oppressed by doubt and depression, but remember that such are not of ourselves, for our Souls know only joy and happiness.

[C.W.,151]

Those who are liable to times of gloom, or even despair, as though a dark cloud overshadowed them and hid the light and the joy of life. It may not be possible to give any reason or explanation for such attacks.

    Under these conditions it is almost impossible to appear happy or cheerful.

[Twelve Healers]

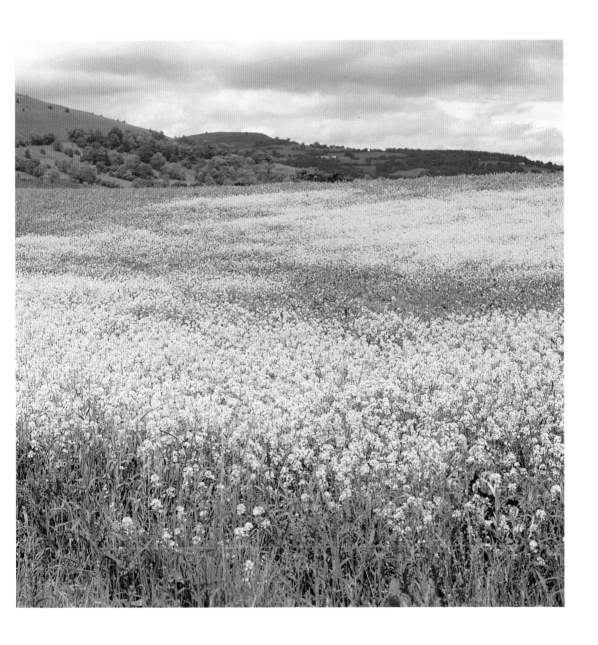

Mustard *Sinapis arvensis*

In recent years we have become familiar with the bright yellow fields of Oil-seed Rape that farmers are growing in many parts of the country. This is *not* the Mustard flower that Bach chose as a remedy for gloom and depression but we may get a feeling for how he saw Mustard growing in arable fields in the 1930s. A sixteenth century herbal speaks of Mustard (or Charlock as it is commonly called) as an 'yll wede' that grows in corn. So it has been a persistent weed on arable land for many generations. Until the advent of selective weedkillers it was difficult to eradicate and was commonly seen to colour whole acres, smothering the planted crops of corn, turnips or grass.

The yellow flower represents cheerfulness, a positive life-affirming brightness, rather as the yellow Gorse does. But Mustard is the remedy for inexplicable depression, the dark mental cloud that appears for no reason. This aspect of the remedy can be recognized in the habit that Mustard has of appearing suddenly, the seeds germinating when the ground has been disturbed. It may be the result of ploughing or road construction. Mustard seeds lie dormant in the soil for many years in what is termed a natural seed bank: hundreds, thousands of seeds may be buried in a square metre of ground waiting their opportunity to grow when conditions are right. When ploughing or digging brings some of them to the right level below the surface they spring up and quickly dominate whatever else may be struggling to cover the bare earth. Thus a Mustard depression often has a link to circumstances in the long past of the soul's life history. The Mustard state of mind, like the plant, is opportunistic—it is a pattern that occupies a vacant space. While the negative form of the remedy state is desolate and in a brown despair, like the bare earth, the positive form of the flower is happy and joyful. The sight of Mustard growing in a field may enrage the farmer but it brightens the land like sunshine.

Locality – Mustard is a common weed on arable land throughout Britain causing considerable problems for farmers; consequently it is being cut, sprayed and generally attacked. But since it reappears everytime the soil is disturbed it is not too difficult to find. It is most commonly seen on the verges of new roads. It avoids acid soils.

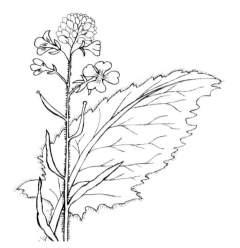 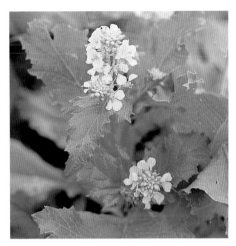

Left: a flowering stalk, with seed pods and leaf.   *Right:* a Mustard plant.

Identification – Mustard is an annual growing up to 50-70 cm. The flowerhead is similar to many other related plants in the cabbage family with yellow four-petalled flowers 15-20 mm. The leaves are dark green, irregularly lobed and toothed, both stem and leaves are hairy. The flowerheads shoot from the axils of the leaves; as flowers open progressively along the stem the seed pods form below. Care is required for identification: most alternatives are hairless, with lighter coloured leaves which have symmetrical lobes.

Flowering Period – Mustard flowers from May through to July.

Preparation – Mustard is prepared by the boiling method (see p.20). Pick the flowerheads above any seed pods when they are blooming strongly early in summer. Collect from as many different plants as possible.

OAK

Our whole object is to realize our faults, and endeavour so to develop the opposing virtue that the faults will disappear from us like snow melts in the sunshine. Don't fight your worries: don't struggle with your disease: don't grapple with your infirmities: rather forget them in concentrating on the development of the virtue you require.

[C.W., 121]

INDICATION

For those who are struggling and fighting strongly to get well, or in connection with the affairs of their daily life. They will go on trying one thing after another, though their case may seem hopeless.

They will fight on. They are discontented with themselves if illness interferes with their duties, or helping others.

They are brave people, fighting against great difficulties, without loss of hope or effort.

[Twelve Healers]

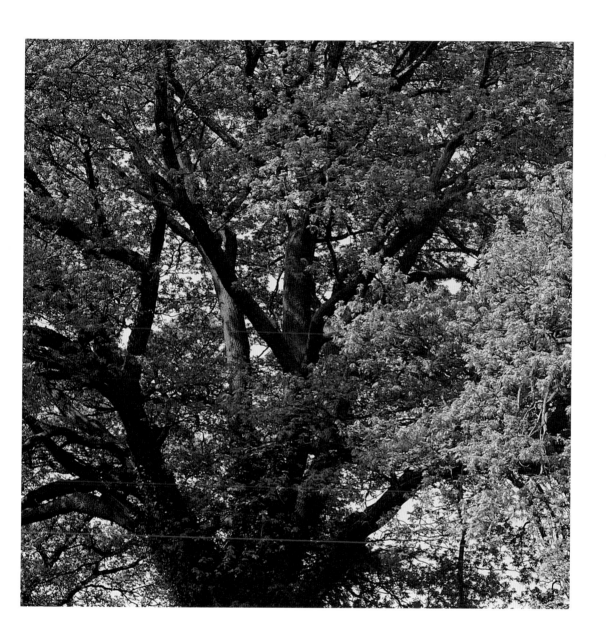

Oak *Quercus robur*

So much tradition surrounds the English Oak—it is characteristic of England being the native forest tree, the emblem of the English yeomen with their reliable and trusted strength. This is the king of trees, the sacred tree of the Druids, the tree that was used to build the ships of the English navy, the great cathedrals, churches and halls. It is a sturdy tree (*robur* means sturdy) mighty and broad, it is rigid and inflexible and will not bend with the wind, yet it is the tree that endures, steadfast and true. All this gives a clue to the nature of the Oak remedy state for these people are like the tree. Like the Oaks they shelter others: in an oakwood many more plants and creatures are to be found than in a beechwood for instance. The Oaks tolerantly host hundreds of different insects, they provide food for the birds and rodents, pannage for the pigs in olden times; they are rich in undergrowth since Oak trees allow light through to the other plants beneath; mosses and even seedling trees grow on their branches. So too the Oak people readily share another's burdens and help to sustain their companions with their own reserves of strength and fortitude.

For all the strength of the Oak tree, however, it is noticeable that they can crack open, branches can break or die back. But Oak trees seem never to give up: they still can be struggling into leaf when the tree is rotten with age. They don't know when to give up, they don't know *how* to give up. So too the Oak person will struggle on with a chronic disability or illness, never accepting defeat. If this is the English Oak we might think of the Englishman's stiff upper lip that never betrays any emotional difficulty, the people who keep on with their daily duty however much they may be suffering. This unwillingness to display weakness is seen also in the hollow trunk of the old Oak. The dead branches are a sign of the tendency of the Oak type to come eventually to breakdown and to a condition 'where the patient loses control over parts of the body or its functions' as Bach described it *[C.W., 72]*. The positive Oak state allows for a more balanced view and an acceptance of limitation, a sharing of the burden and the development of less rigid ways to express the will.

Locality – Oaks grow throughout Britain. Sessile Oaks predominate in the north and west on the poorer soils while *Q. robur* is more common in the south-east of the country.

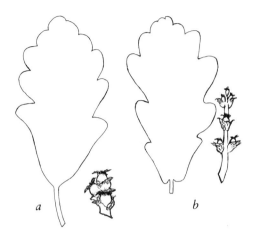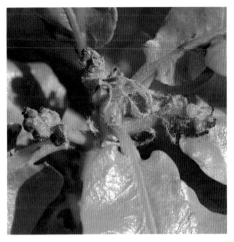

Left: leaves and flowers of (a) Sessile Oak (b) Pedunculate Oak. **Right:** *detail of the female flowers.*

Identification – There are many varieties of Oak in the northern hemisphere but only two native British Oaks: the English or Pedunculate Oak (*Q. robur*) and the Sessile or Durmast Oak (*Q. petraea*). In general appearance they are similar although the Sessile Oak tends to grow taller with a more slender unbranched trunk. The important distinction lies in the flower and leaf. The English Oak (Bach's remedy Oak) has leaves with little or no stalk (ironically this is technically Sessile) and female flowers (and later acorns) that are on stalks or peduncles 20-30 mm long. The Sessile Oak conversely has stalked leaves and unstalked (sessile) female flowers. These female flowers in both cases are like small, red buds. The male flowers are catkins that hang like knotted string (25-45 mm) from the ends of the branches. The female flowers appear on the new season's growth right at the end of the twigs. As it is difficult to pick the flowers of the Sessile Oak, the English Oak with a stalked flower is the one to use.

Flowering Period – during late April and May. The flowers appear with the new leaves when they are ochre in colour before they darken to green.

Preparation – Oak is prepared by the sun method (see p.20). Choose a place near an oakwood with an open southern aspect and gather the red female flowers only from as many trees as possible. Pick the whole stalk of flowers and float them on to the water so as to cover the surface.

OLIVE

We each have a Divine mission in this world, and our souls use our minds and bodies as instruments to do this work, so that when all three are working in unison the result is perfect health and perfect happiness.

[C.W., 91]

Those who have suffered much mentally or physically and are so exhausted and weary that they feel they have no more strength to make any effort. Daily life is hard work for them, without pleasure.

[Twelve Healers]

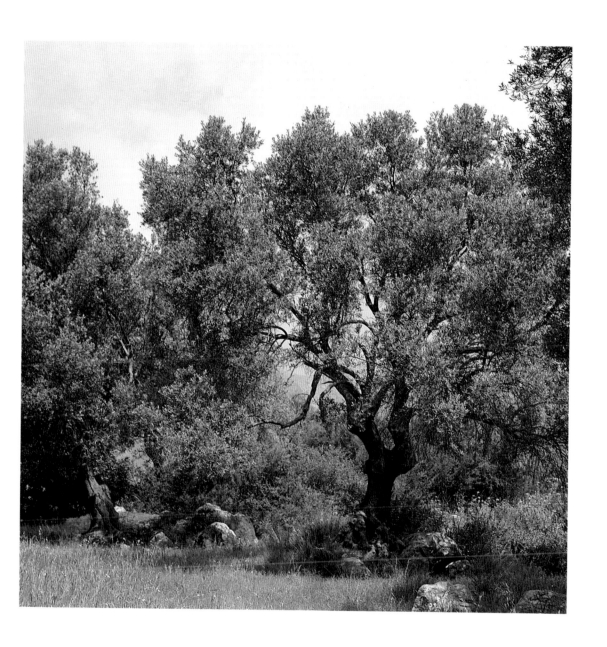

Olive *Olea europaea*

The Olive is a native of the hot Mediterranean lands. With little water and burned by the sun it is a stunted tree, slow growing and long lived. It has been cultivated since ancient times for the fruit and the oil that is extracted from it. Olive is one of the seven remedies which Bach said were for chronic conditions when people had been ill for months or even years. Like the Vine (see p.148), another of the *Seven Helpers*, we are told that it survived the Great Flood along with Noah since the last dove that he sent out flew back with an Olive branch. Hence the Olive tree has become a symbol of peace, reconciliation and renewal. The remedy state of Olive describes those who are worn out and exhausted after much worry, illness, grief or some long struggle. After his ordeal in the ark which lasted for just over a year Noah may well have felt as if he had no strength to carry on! Just so it was to the Mount of Olives that Jesus went on the night that he was arrested to be taken before Pilate. These trees had the essential vitality that helped to renew his strength; meanwhile his weary companions had fallen asleep.

To set Olive in a modern context, it is the remedy for those who have suffered from burn-out, when their reserves of energy are so drained by the demands of helping others that they have nothing left for themselves. In the same way the Olive tree gives unstintingly, generation after generation. It continues to flower even in extremity, when bent and hollow with age; in its last year it will give fruit. These old trees are often cut to a stump and then they start anew with three or four young stems growing up from the old wood. Olive trees are apparently inexhaustible. It is a part of their strength that they can help those who are exhausted, giving them support and comfort.

Locality – Olive trees are native to the Mediterranean. The remedy essence is not made in Britain; Bach mentions Italy but any country where wild Olive trees are found will serve. Commercial Olive groves, which overwork the land, are not suitable. It is better to go into the mountains. Where there is is a great variety of wild flowers you have the assurance of healthy and strong land. These photographs were taken in Crete.

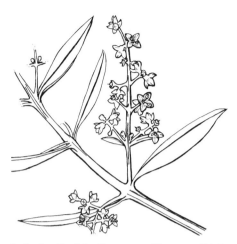 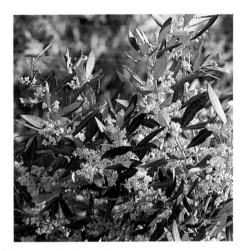

Left: detail of the flowers and leaves. ***Right:*** *detail of the flowering branches.*

Identification – Olive is a small tree of 5-15 m with pale grey bark, much branched, with grey-green foliage. The leaves are silvery beneath and leathery, 45-60 mm long, in opposite pairs. The flowers grow along a stem (in racemes) which springs from the axil of the leaf, twenty or more flowers together on each raceme. Each individual flower is small with four creamy white petals.

Flowering Period – this varies according to locality and season but it is generally in May or June.

Preparation – Olive is prepared by the sun method (see p.20). The flowering clusters are picked when in perfect bloom from as many trees as possible. Float them on to the water so as to cover the surface.

PINE

Health is, therefore, the true realization of what we are: we are perfect: we are the children of God. There is no striving to gain what we have already attained. We are merely here to manifest in material form the perfection with which we have been endowed from the beginning of time.

[C.W., 92]

INDICATION

For those who blame themselves. Even when successful they think they could have done better, and are never content with their efforts or the results. They are hard-working and suffer much from the faults they attach to themselves.

Sometimes if there is any mistake it is due to another, but they will claim responsibility even for that.

[Twelve Healers]

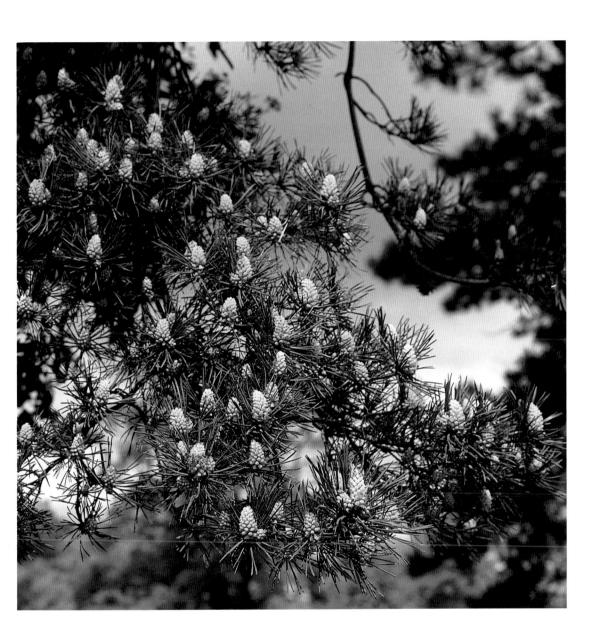

Pine *Pinus sylvestris*

If we go to look at Pine trees two things are particularly striking: first the straightness of the growth and the pointed, needle leaves, secondly the aromatic smell. These characteristics made the Pine tree important commercially for its straight-grained timber and the oils of turpentine. The scent of Pine is well known and comes from the resinous sap that exudes through the bark. It has a penetrating clarity with great cleansing properties; its sharpness acts to clear obstructions and straighten out entanglement. This applies both physically and emotionally. As a flower remedy Pine is concerned with feelings of guilt, blame and a sense of failing to live up to expectation. The emotional responses are entangled and confused by past experiences so that we do not see what is really going on. Often this is not just a temporary condition when we blame ourselves for a specific failure or mistake, rather it is a deep-seated attitude to life that has developed over a long period. When the flower essence is made it shows an interesting reflection of this as it has a taste like stale, dry lumber, something old and fusty. Pine acts to clear old emotional knots and tease out the confused pattern of self-reproach.

The feeling of guilt can sometimes be linked to a childhood in which a parent was cruelly dominant. Children that are always 'told off' and treated severely can grow to anticipate angry punishment and then come to assume guilt even when they are entirely without blame. As adults they are unable to see emotional situations clearly; they cannot tell what is their responsibility and what is the responsibility of another. The positive form of the Pine state is seen in the loving parent who assists us to develop our individuality in accordance with the dictates of our inner being. Like a comb it separates the tangled strands that have caused us emotional confusion leaving us with a clear, balanced and objective view of our involvement with life. We learn to accept that we are beloved, that we are safe, that we are supported. The straightness of the Pine at our back gives strength and clarity to the heart.

Locality – Pines grow throughout Britain, often on the poorer thin soils, on gravel and greensand.

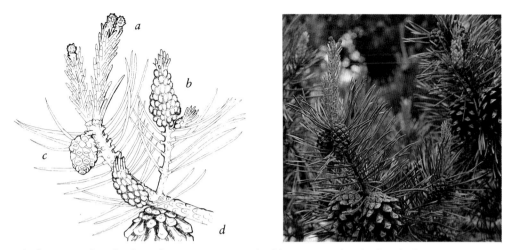

Left: flowers (a) female, (b) male; (c) young cone (d) old cone.   *Right:* the female flowers.

Identification – Pine trees are tall evergreens growing up to 35 m high. The leaves of *P. sylvestris* are clusters of paired needles 50-75 mm, shorter than some other Pines. Male and female flowers are on the same tree; males are a cluster of small yellow balls at the base of the new shoot; females are red, cone-shaped and appear at the end of the new growth. All the Pines display a kind of continuous growth with old cones ripening as new ones form. Altogether some fifty varieties can be found listed in a book on trees—a simple identification is not possible. The differences can often be detected in the cone but the general form of the tree is a good guide: the Scots Pine, which Bach chose, has the characteristic head of branches on a pale rust coloured trunk.

Flowering Period – May.

Preparation – Pine is prepared by the boiling method (see p.20). Both male and females flowers are gathered from several different trees, on twigs about 15 cm long so as to fit the saucepan. The remedy should be made when the male flowers are mature: shake the branch gently and you will see a cloud of yellow pollen if the time is right.

RED CHESTNUT

Everyone of us also has sympathy with those in distress, and naturally so, because we have all been in distress ourselves at some time in our lives. So that not only can we heal ourselves, but we have the great privilege of being able to help others to heal themselves, and the only qualifications necessary are love and sympathy.

[C.W., 99]

INDICATION

For those who find it difficult not to be anxious for other people.

    Often they have ceased to worry about themselves, but for those of whom they are fond they may suffer much, frequently anticipating that some unfortunate thing may happen to them.

[Twelve Healers]

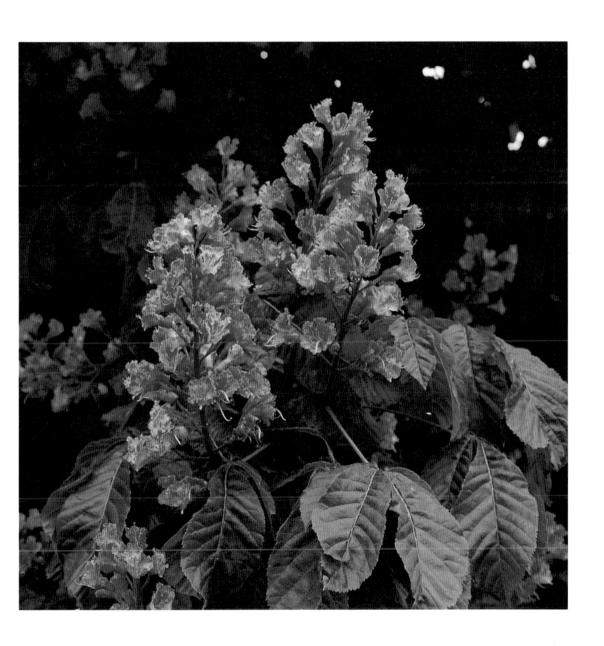

Red Chestnut   *Aesculus Carnea*

In an emergency, or even when there is just the possibility of something going wrong, our thoughts will influence the situation. If, in our minds, we anticipate misfortune then we help to create the pattern that brings misfortune about. For this reason Bach sought a remedy that would calm the mind of those who projected fear, so that they might have harmonious rather than disruptive thoughts. Other remedies, such as Holly or Impatiens, can be seen to calm those who are pushing out their negativity. But Red Chestnut is concerned specifically with the projection of fear and anxiety, not on our own account, but as fear for the well-being of others. This can manifest as worrying about the ones we love.

When the Red Chestnut is in bloom with the whole tree full of deep pink-red flowers it radiates a clear, warm strength that is both loving (in the pink) and powerful (in the red). The sight of the flowers as a mass of small starbursts expresses both the projected energy and the diffused worrying quality of this remedy state. The radiating force is made stronger in the Red Chestnut by the contrasting dark green of the leaves. They are a complement to the red and this causes a strong optical vibration.

The Red Chestnut tree is apparently the result of a chance hybrid between the Horse Chestnut (*A. hippocastanum*) and the American Red Buckeye (*A. pavia*). Botanists are unsure as to why this cross should remain and breed true as a new species and speak of a spontaneous doubling of the chromosomes. It first appeared about 1820 and is widely planted for its ornamental colour. It is not a strong tree and lacks a certain vitality, being subject to inexplicable decay. That weakness is also part of its nature and offers an insight into the fear state that the tree embodies. Red Chestnut people have a gentle softness like the tree. But the strength of the colour in the flowers supports them so that they come to radiate confidence in life and happiness.

Locality – Red Chestnut trees are generally found throughout Britain. They are often planted in avenues and groups where they show their colour to advantage. They rarely grow wild.

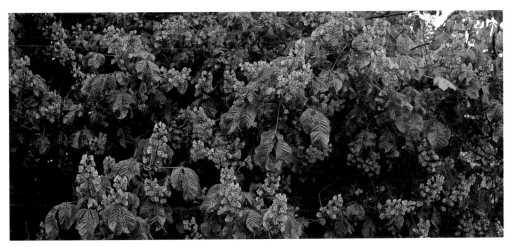
Red Chestnut in flower.

Identification – Red Chestnut is easy to recognize, it grows 10-15m high, smaller in all respects than the White or Horse Chestnut (see p.160). The trunk is furrowed and the bark broken; the branches tend to be light, slender and drooping. The buds (see Chestnut Bud p.48) are brown, tinged with green-purple; the dark green leaves are palmate, having between five and seven leaflets radiating from a single stalk. The flowers form an erect cluster at the end of the branch along a stem of 10-20 cm. The individual red flowers are some 10-20 mm across.

Flowering Period – late May and June, a little later than the White Chestnut.

Preparation – Red Chestnut is prepared by the boiling method (see p.20). The flowering spurs are picked in full flower from as many different trees as possible.

ROCK ROSE

All fear must be cast out; it should never exist in the human mind, and is only possible when we lose sight of our Divinity. It is foreign to us because as Sons of the Creator, Sparks of the Divine Life, we are invincible, indestructible and unconquerable.

[C.W., 155]

INDICATION

The rescue remedy. The remedy of emergency for cases where there even appears no hope. In accidents or sudden illness, or when the patient is very frightened or terrified, or if the condition is serious enough to cause great fear to those around. If the patient is not conscious the lips may be moistened with the remedy. Other remedies in addition may also be required, as, for example, if there is unconsciousness, which is a deep, sleepy state, Clematis; if there is torture, Agrimony, and so on.

[Twelve Healers]

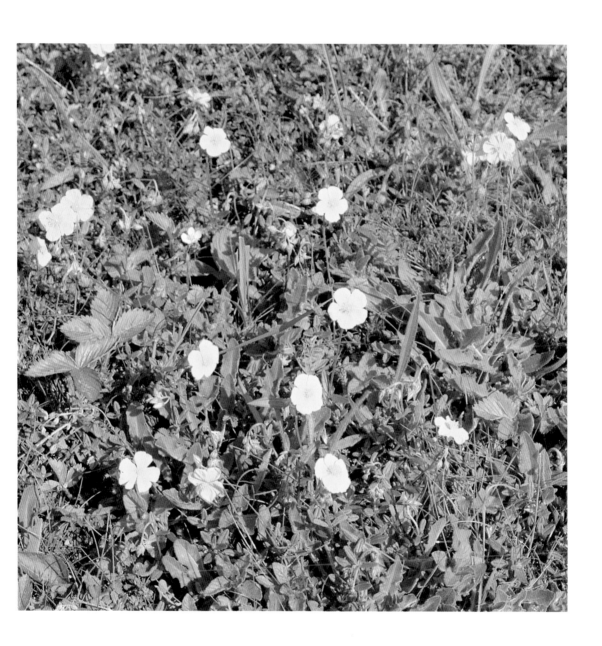

Rock Rose *Helianthemum nummularium*

The botanical name given to the Common Rock Rose—*Helianthemum nummularium*—derives from the Greek *Helios*, sun, and the Latin word for coins, suggesting the pure golden flowers that shine like golden coins in the sunshine. We all know the buttercup and dandelion but yellow though they are they seem almost dull compared to the Rock Rose which has a startling radiance. The clear brightness of the colour is displayed in large, open, flat petals that form the disc of the coin. The central part of the flower too radiates the golden yellow in the numerous stamens. Growing in short grass on the hillside it can form a carpet of brightness that absorbs and reflects back the pure life-light of the sun. It is simply this that makes Rock Rose so potent as a healer.

The Rock Rose remedy state describes the panic, terror and despair that can grip people in an emergency. Bach spoke of it as the rescue remedy. He said it was to bring courage to win through against great odds, when we find ourselves in a 'fight for mental freedom' *[C.W., 80]*. This refers to the need for mental clarity when our emotions are in a state of chaotic fear. Again the colour of the flower denotes this: bright yellow reflects clear thought and gold is the colour of radiant steadiness in the heart. Just as it is the strong clear light of the sun that disperses mist so the golden Rock Rose clears the grey clouds of fear. It brings a peace and tranquillity to those caught up in an emergency. Looking at the flower with its frail petals we can feel a quiet reverence. Amid the urgency of terror this plant reminds us of those forces that are eternal, beyond the vibratory and changing. Bach thought this would be an experience of the essential knowledge and truth which would remove all fear from our minds. Lacking that realization we must struggle on, yet, as he says, 'it may be part of the Divine Plan that we prove ourselves far greater by battling on, though we are afraid; and it is for mankind to discover the way to see the Light and remove from mankind the burden of fear.' *[C.W., 26]*

Locality – Rock Rose is found in southern England in upland pastures on dry, rocky soils, generally on chalk.

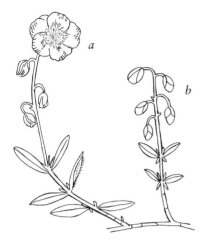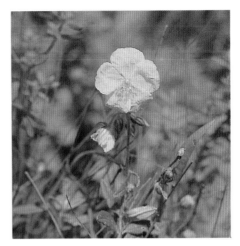

Left: the trailing stems with (a) flower (b) buds.   *Right:* detail of the flowers.

Identification – Rock Rose is a small perennial plant with trailing branches which send up short erect stems with a head of drooping flower buds. The flowers open one or two at a time with five bright yellow petals 20-25mm across, which soon fade and die. Leaves are in opposite pairs, lanceolate and hairy, downy white beneath; small leaf-like stipules spring from the base of each leaf. Once recognized Rock Rose will not be confused with other plants, but it is worth mentioning that a trailing buttercup has a cup-shaped flower while Rock Rose is flat and larger. Cinquefoils too have a smaller flower and a very different leaf.

Flowering Period – late May through to August.

Preparation – Rock Rose is prepared by the sun method (see p.20). Choose a place where the plant grows strongly and gather the single flowers from several different clumps, floating them on the surface of the water. Dr Bach mentions specifically that while garden varieties may exist only those growing in the wild should be used for preparing the essence.

ROCK WATER

This remedy brings great peace and understanding, broadens the outlook that all people must find perfection in their own individual way, and brings the realization of 'being' and not 'doing'; of being in ourselves a reflection of Great Things and not attempting to put forward our own ideas.

[C.W., 73]

INDICATION

Those who are very strict in their way of living; they deny themselves many of the joys and pleasures of life because they consider it might interfere with their work.

They are hard masters to themselves. They wish to be well and strong and active, and will do anything which they believe will keep them so. They hope to be examples which will appeal to others who may then follow their ideas and be better as a result.

[Twelve Healers]

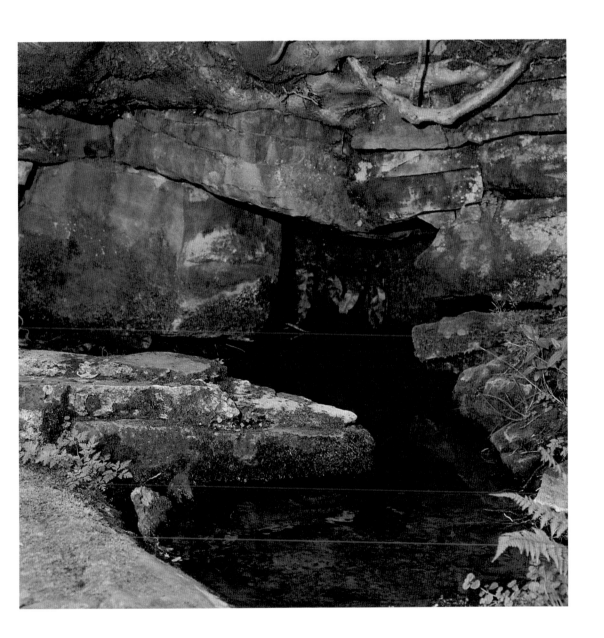

Rock Water

Our planet, the earth, is a living being. It moves, breathes (one full breath every twenty-four hours with the respiration of the plants), it has systems to circulate its life force and fluids and, if we choose to think of it as a body, it has what appears to be a nervous system with some areas that we feel to be charged and sensitive. The complexity of this being is little understood by us even though we live in its surface. At school we learned that water in the sea is caught up from the waves' crest by the wind, taken to the land and cast down as rain. Percolating through the rock it springs out to form the source for first, a mountain stream, which becomes a brook, then a river, which in time flows back to the sea. Physical science can measure the way in which this whole process cleanses the water but it also has a metaphysical action that is part of the life of the planet. This renews, refines and recharges the water. It is most vital not when it is in the sea, nor in the rain but when it first springs from the inside of the earth. It was from natural spring water that Bach made the remedy Rock Water, in 1933, at the same time that he was in Wales to prepare the essence of Heather. Interestingly, he spent the last years of his life in the village of *Sotwell* living at a house called *The Wellsprings*.

Rock Water is for people in whom idealism has become fanatical so that they live by strict theories rather than the gentle acceptance of experience. The soft, pure water of the earth helps to soften the rigidity of this mentality, even as running water will wear away a stone. Yet this Rock Water is not made from just any well. It also derives its properties from the innate healing qualities of the chosen place, where the concentration of earth forces charge that location. Such places are usually known as holy or marked by the names of saints, people whose lives were pure and who were an example to their contemporaries. This is what the Rock Water person would like to be. The purity that they seek in themselves is indeed found in the true purity of the water. In the positive of this remedy state we can come to learn inwardly that all must flow with the lessons of life: water takes the line of least resistance. Water can adapt by responding to change while it is the stone that is set in its way. It is all there, mirrored in the earth, an object lesson for mankind, an allegory for our quest.

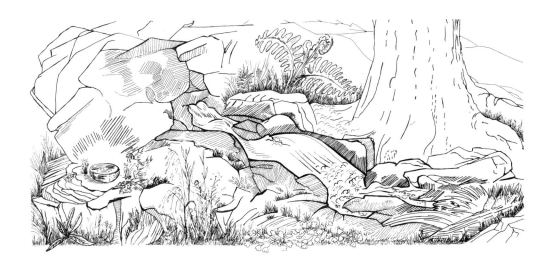

Locality – Bach's own instructions are quite clear:

> It has long been known that certain well- and spring-waters have had the power to heal a limited number of people, and such wells or springs have become renowned for this property. Any well or spring which has been known to be a healing centre and which is still left free in its natural state, unhampered by the shrines of man, may be used. *[C.W., 74]*.

Many attractive sites should be avoided simply because they are well known or the flow of water has been channelled or controlled. The source should be protected by natural forces but unfettered by man. The photograph is of St Thomas' Well in Herefordshire.

Identification – There are a great number of holy wells in Britain (and elsewhere) and a local map will often mark the sites. On seeing a well it may at once be apparent if it is either disturbed, polluted or interfered with. Often they are lost in a field but then there can be the problem of cattle or sheep or chemicals from farming which seep into the water table. It is important to find one that still has pure water and that will probably mean going to high ground; nuclear fall-out will also be a problem in parts of the country. Common sensitivity will make a good choice.

Preparation – Rock Water is prepared by the sun method (see p.20). Choose a perfect day in midsummer and simply expose the bowl of water in clear sunlight. Bach mentions that one hour is sufficient to make the remedy but a longer time may be advisable.

SCLERANTHUS

AFFIRMATION

Instability can be eradicated by the development of self-determination, by making up the mind and doing things with definiteness instead of wavering and hovering. Even if at first we may sometimes make errors, it were better to act than to let opportunities pass for want of a decision. Determination will soon grow; fear of plunging into life will disappear, and the experiences gained will guide our mind to better judgement.

[C.W., 136]

INDICATION

Those who suffer much from being unable to decide between two things, first one seeming right then the other.

They are usually quiet people, and bear their difficulty alone, as they are not inclined to discuss it with others.

[Twelve Healers]

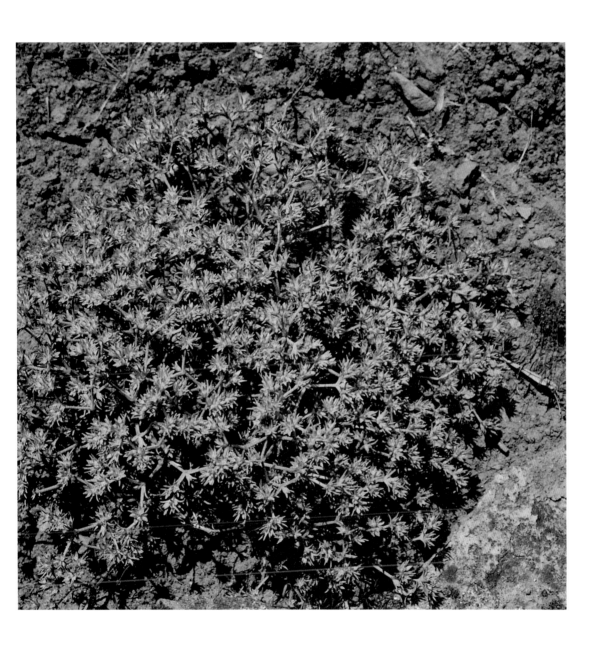

Scleranthus   *Scleranthus annuus*

The Scleranthus remedy state describes a kind of mental uncertainty, a yes/no ambivalence about life. It is said that we were born on earth because of our desire for life and in the negative of this remedy state the desire is confused. This shows as a changeableness physically, emotionally and mentally. A Scleranthus person lacks the central point of reference, the ego-ism, that directs the life towards ordinary selfish ends, consequently they cannot make up their minds. So the positive of this remedy requires more than a new colouring of the emotions, it needs, rather, a re-forming of the link to our inner being, the consciousness of our Self. This is illustrated in the fact that the flower, unusually, has no petals. Other plants act to receive and broadcast the force patterns of particular emotional states through the colour that we perceive in their petals. This plant, however, acts from a slightly different level. Some of the other Bach flowers such as Wild Oat (see p.164) also lack petals and they share certain qualities.

Scleranthus is an inconspicuous plant that is easily overlooked. Where it was found last week it may be gone today, eaten by rabbits or burned off by the sun. In the grass it can be seen one moment and then apparently disappear the next. Once found it is evident and known; this too points to its nature. Like morality it is implicit but hard to define. Its common name of Knawel derives from the German for a knot or tangled threads. The tangled stems of the plant, which seem to grow in all directions at once, bespeak a need for clarity and discrimination. The colour of the flowers, green, suggests that it will be provided by an insight of the heart. Those of us who lack conviction are finding the way to a new perception, a new way to make up the mind. This will be more than a choice between left and right, coming or going. There is a discrimination of the soul that can direct our actions by the conviction of a deeper purpose. It is to this that the humble Scleranthus bears witness, bringing a clear and open perception of what is most appropriate.

Locality – Scleranthus grows on sandy soil (not calcareous), in dry or well drained conditions. Bach and the authors of some early *Floras* list it as common, notably in cornfields. But with modern agricultural practices it has become quite scarce and being small it is difficult to find in any case. It will be found growing on uncultivated land where natural grazing has broken the surface of the ground. This may be done by rabbits, who also like sandy soil for their burrows!

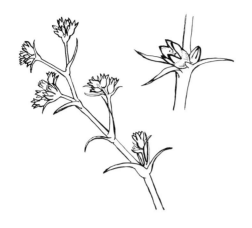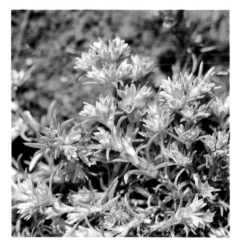

Left: a single flowering stem.   *Right: detail of the flowering plant.*

Identification – Scleranthus is an annual (the Perennial Knawel is similar but woody). It grows low on the ground with numerous branched stems that form in a tangled cushion. The leaves are small and spiky, clasping the stem in pairs. The cluster of flowers at the end of the shoots are green, 4mm across and without petals. The five pointed sepals might be mistaken for petals. They give the appearance of a tiny crown. The fruit is a dry nut that forms in the centre. A search for Scleranthus may lead to many similar plants being found: some of the Spurreys and Pearlworts in particular might be taken in error. Procumbent Pearlwort (*Sagina Procumbens*) grows where Scleranthus will not, in damp and shaded places.

Flowering Period – late May to September.

Preparation – Scleranthus is prepared by the sun method (see p.20). Find a place where the plant grows strongly and pick the flowering heads floating them on to the surface of the water. This may involve picking some seeds so the Scleranthus can be helped by seeing them safely back on to the earth when the essence has been made.

STAR of BETHLEHEM

...to remain in such a state of peace that the trials and disturbances of the world leave us unruffled, is a great attainment indeed and brings to us that Peace which passeth understanding; and though at first it may seem to be beyond our dreams, it is in reality, with patience and perseverence, within the reach of us all.

[C.W., 153]

INDICATION

For those in distress under conditions which for a time produce great unhappiness.

The shock of serious news, the loss of someone dear, the fright following an accident, and such like.

For those who for a time refuse to be consoled this remedy brings comfort.

[Twelve Healers]

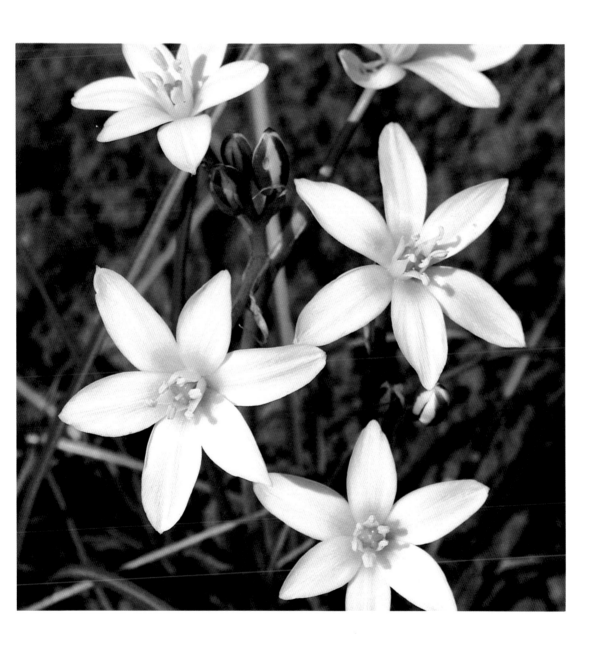

Star of Bethlehem   *Ornitholagum umbellatum*

Star of Bethlehem is a six-petalled flower. Like the Star of David, this star has an especial meaning. The name also relates to the fact that a plant of this kind grows profusely in the fields of Palestine and Syria. The stars of those lands have some obvious associations. This small flower that shines with an intense whiteness, displays a perfect six-fold geometry. In the natural world geometry has a wondrous meaning. It was only in quite recent times that the *Mogen David* became the symbol of Judaism. It was used in antiquity because it demonstrated the idea that life was due to the interpenetration of matter and Divinity: one triangle representing the Divine world touching to earth, the other the material world reaching towards God. When they are in perfect relationship a perfect attunement exists in life. If they are out of kilter, however, it is easy to see that all things would be displaced and out of harmony. As this is the only one of the Bach flowers that has this six-fold geometry (most of them are five-fold) it has a particular significance.

Star of Bethlehem is for shock. When we suffer a shock of any kind it has the tendency to drive us out of our bodies—we say 'I jumped out of my skin...' or 'it knocked me sideways...'. We have a picture then of the dislocation of the subtle geometry of ourselves: we are out of balance. This distorts the flow of the life force within us and has serious effects upon our health at all levels. Star of Bethlehem has the strength in its bright radiant purity to realign the pattern. It acts to unify us again so that the natural healing processes can take place. In practical terms we feel comforted and soothed so that our pain and trauma is eased; we find that we can breathe again and release tension. That is to say a state of normal activity can resume because the harmony of our divine nature is again in place.

Locality – Star of Bethlehem grows in open grassland on drier soils. It is not uncommon but is most likely to be found in the south and east of England. Old flower books speak of it as being an introduced species to be found in cottage gardens, though if it is not a native species it has generally naturalized.

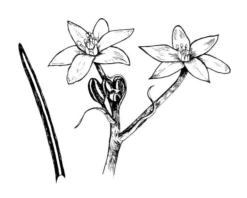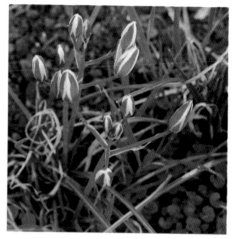

Left: flowers with leaf and buds. **Right:** *closed flowers have a green stripe on the back of the petals.*

Identification – Star of Bethlehem is a perennial bulb of the Lily family. When in flower it has a stem and leaves of about 10-15 cm. The leaves are slender and pointed, growing from the bulb, dark green with a white central vein. The flowers are held in an umbel—a head of between six and ten separately stemmed flowers—each flower (30mm across) having six petals. These are bright white with a dark green stripe on the back; this is due to their dual function as sepals forming a green bud before opening. Within the six petals is a central coronet of six stamens, very pronounced, raised on white stalks surrounding a central dome. The flowers are displayed to gain maximum light and open fully only in bright sunshine. The plant is easily recognized though some of its relatives might mislead: Ramsons, wild garlic, for instance has a broad leaf and a flowerhead of plain white stars, while others have a distinctly different structure.

Flowering Period – April to June.

Preparation – Star of Bethlehem is prepared by the boiling method (see p.20). Find a place where the plant is prolific and pick the flowerheads complete. The flowers should be open so a bright, clear morning is required.

SWEET CHESTNUT

AFFIRMATION

But in the darkest hours, and when success seems well-nigh impossible, let us
ever remember that God's children should never be afraid, that our Souls only
give us such tasks as we are capable of accomplishing, and that with our own
courage and faith in the Divinity within us victory must come to all who continue
to strive.

[C.W., 141]

INDICATION

For those moments which happen to some people when the anguish is so great
as to seem to be unendurable.

When the mind or body feels as if it had borne to the uttermost limit of its
endurance, and that now it must give way.

When it seems there is nothing but destruction and annihilation left to face.

[Twelve Healers]

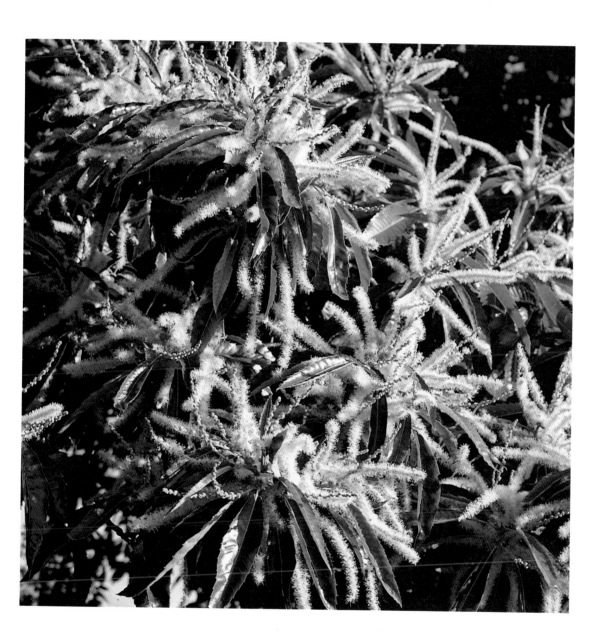

Sweet Chestnut *Castanea sativa*

Among the last of the series of the flower remedies that Bach found was the Sweet Chestnut. This was to be for the feelings of anguish and despair. We might wonder what kind of a flower would have the strength to help us through what seems unendurable, when the soul is desolate. Surely a tree with the utmost strength and vitality would be needed. It is a time when we feel that we face annihilation, when we feel that mentally we can go no further, we can suffer no more. Sweet Chestnuts are among the most magnificent of trees. They grow to be huge with a powerful self-contained quality, a solitary presence of great and sufficient strength. They can live more than a thousand years and, like the positive aspect of the remedy that leads to new insight and new possibilities, the old trees can begin new growth from the old trunk. They demonstrate a life force that is quite exceptional, capable of carrying aloft into the sunlight the exhausted spirit of those who have wrestled in the darkness below.

In winter the vast trunks rise straight and sheer with a strong and undiffused force which can be seen in the rippling of the bark, which is combed with vertical furrows along its length. These furrows often show a spiralling around the trunk, a pattern that may denote the presence of a particular focus of earth forces. In summer the trunk is obscured by the dense foliage, the leaves large, tough and shiny with wax. The explosion of flowers that covers the whole tree in July is the climax of its powerful thrust into life.

The Sweet or Spanish Chestnut, like the Olive, (see p.112) is a native of southern Europe. It is thought to have been brought to England by the Romans. Being a Mediterranean tree it enjoys hot and direct sun. This suggests the strength it has to warm the heart and straighten the bowed spirit: its gesture being to look up and out. The flowers show this too in their creamy plumes that appear like trailing bursts of warm light.

Locality – Sweet Chestnut grows in many parts of Britain although only in the south does it do well and seed itself into the wild. Elsewhere specimens have been planted as ornaments in parkland. It prefers a light and well-drained soil (especially sand) but it is tolerant of most conditions except for lime.

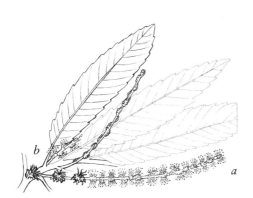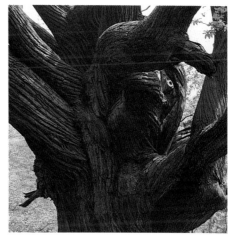

Left: flowers (a) male, (b) female.   ***Right:*** *the massive trunk of an old tree.*

Identification – Sweet Chestnut is not difficult to recognize. It grows about 30 m or more in height, not the tallest of trees but with great stature. Mature specimens show a girth of 10 m in England and considerably more further south. The furrowed bark is characteristic, the long, pointed leaves (15-25 cm) are dark green, shiny with coarsely toothed edges. The trees are known for the edible nuts produced in autumn inside a prickly case. These come from the female flowers that are not conspicuous compared with the showy plumes of the male catkins. The males are 20-25 cm long with groups of fifty or more delicate stamens, creamy-gold. The green female flowers are either at the bottom of the male stalk or separate in the axil of the flowering shoot. They are formed into a cup by four bracts with a divided seed chamber and tufted style.

Flowering Period – usually after midsummer, in July.

Preparation – Sweet Chestnut is prepared by the boiling method (see p.20). Pick the flowering heads when they are well in bloom, the male flowers being creamy yellow. Both male and female flowers are used along with any leaves. Gather from as many different trees as possible although only a few of these flowering heads will fit into the saucepan.

VERVAIN

We should strive to be so gentle, so quiet, so patiently helpful that we move among our fellow men more as a breath of air or a ray of sunshine: ever ready to help them when they ask: but never forcing them to our own views.

[C.W., 119]

Those with fixed principles and ideas, which they are confident are right, and which they very rarely change.

They have a great wish to convert all around them to their own views of life.

They are strong of will and have much courage when they are convinced of those things that they wish to teach.

In illness they struggle on long after many would have given up their duties.

[Twelve Healers]

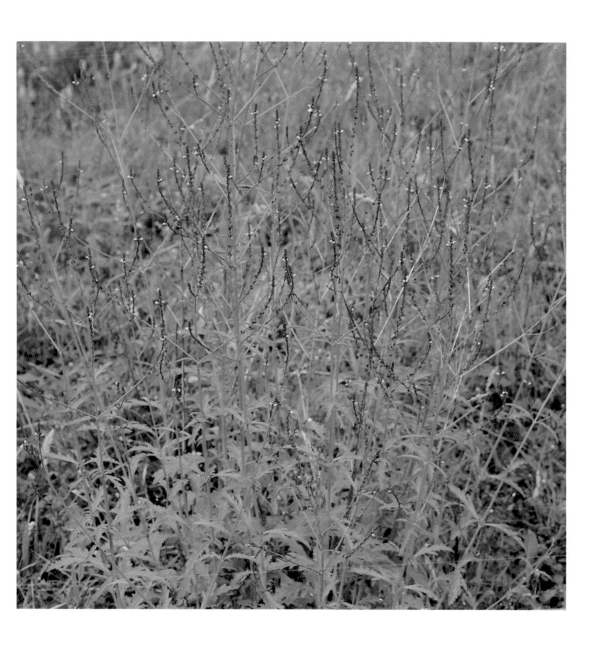

Vervain *Verbena officianalis*

In attempting to understand the nature of the various remedy plants we look at the flowers, their colour and where they grow. We also look at the plant's structure. This gives a first clue to Vervain, the remedy for over-effort and stress. Whilst all plants are perfect there is a feeling that Vervain has got things out of proportion. The flowers are tiny and inconspicuous yet the stems are quite tall and branching, producing a shrubby plant. There are few leaves and they are mostly at the base. So there is a considerable growth of structure, a network of stems, that supports almost nothing; unlike other plants there is no crown of foliage and flowers. Being a Mediterranean herb this may be a way to survive the hot and dry conditions but it also creates a picture of the Vervain remedy state which Bach described as the need 'to realize that the big things in life are done gently and quietly without strain or stress' *[C.W., 107]*. There can be no bigger event for a plant than coming to flower and so achieving an essential life purpose; yet if the stems to carry the buds are overdoing it the Vervain flowers are so modest, gentle and peaceable as to be almost unnoticed. But big ideals can be attained without stress and hurry, without a great display; that is the life lesson of the Vervain.

It is the tranquillity that the flowers embody that carries the essence of the remedy. Their pale mauve colour is calming and if we examine them closely we are drawn into an inner world where conflict, tension and hurry are forgotten. Outwardly the plant shows the frantic jerky growth of the negative state with its restless movement. Inwardly it shows the receptive restraint that balances it, bringing harmony to life. Like the Agrimony type (the structure of the two plants is similar in certain respects, see p.24) the Vervain person essentially seeks peace. Both see that there is much wrong in the world but Agrimony suffers internally while Vervain pushes the conflict outwards. Vervain is concerned with the outer circumstances of life and has the desire to see them changed. Curiously it grows where land has been disturbed and although it likes some shelter it is often seen on the roadside of some new by-pass. As the cars and lorries rush by the tiny star-like flowers call from a distant dimension of calm.

Locality – Vervain grows on bare, dry ground where grass is sparse. Hedges and roadside verges are the most likely sites although the chemical sprays that were used on verges some years ago destroyed many plants. Now it is found on recently cleared ground where competition is not strong. It is rather local, growing mostly in southern England, especially on chalk.

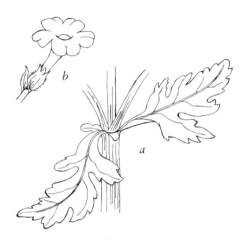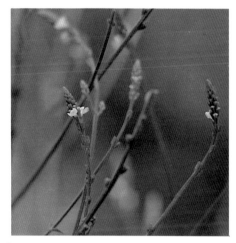

*Left: (a) the stalk and leaves, (b) the structure of a single flower.   **Right:** detail of the flowering stems.*

Identification – Vervain grows up to 1m high from a perennial rootstock with rather strong bushy stems. Last year's dead stalks often remain with the plant. The stems are square in section and like the leaves they are hairy. Leaves are pinnate and opposite, deeply lobed and toothed, being smaller higher up the plant. Flowers are small (4-5mm) pale mauve or pink, opening progressively along a slender spike with small fruits forming below. Only a few flowers open at one time.

Flowering Period – June to September.

Preparation – Vervain is prepared by the sun method (see p.20). The flowering spikes are picked from as many different plants as possible. These are cut above any seeds that have formed when there are several small flowers in bloom. The cut stems are floated on to the bowl of water.

147

VINE

AFFIRMATION

If we set everybody and everything around us at liberty, we find that in return we are richer in love and possessions than ever we were before, for the love that gives freedom is the great love that binds the closer.

[C.W., 103]

INDICATION

Very capable people, certain of their own ability, confident of success.

Being so assured, they think that it would be for the benefit of others if they could be persuaded to do things as they themselves do, or as they are certain is right. Even in illness they will direct their attendants.

They may be of great value in emergency.

[Twelve Healers]

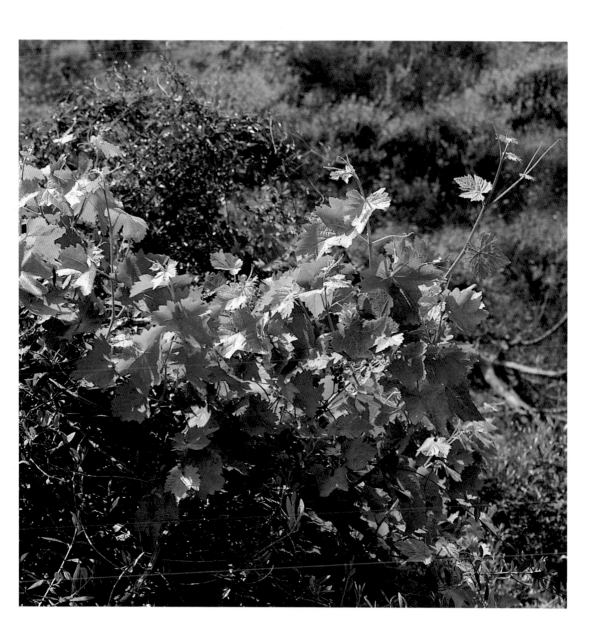

Vine *Vitis vinifera*

The Vine is one of the oldest recorded plants: like the Olive it must have survived the Great Flood for we are told that Noah planted a vineyard. Throughout the Bible the work of growing and dressing vines is used to illustrate the life circumstances of people. The Vine needs careful tending and if wrongly selected may bear bitter and unpalatable fruit. So it came to represent an allegory for the life of the soul. Equally, as a provider of both food and drink the Vine has had a long and unique association with mankind. As a Bach remedy it is the natural behaviour of the wild plant that is important. The pruned and restrained cultivated vine has a twisted and cramped old stock forced by the growers to their demands. Compared to the free stretching of the trailing stalks of the wild variety it is a harsh treatment. Yet both forms of Vine reach out and grip whatever is nearby, twisting the tendrils to fasten hold.

The remedy state is described as domineering, self-willed and inflexible. Bach says that those who dominate require 'much help and guidance to enable them to realize that great universal truth of Unity and to understand the joy of Brotherhood' *[C.W., 141]*. The Vine state loses sight of compassion and fellowship in the sureness of the individual will. It is as if we forget our divine origin and forget that there is divinity in each of us. Thus we can become petty tyrants. Much in the growth of the Vine illustrates this: it is a climber that is extremely strong, with tendrils that bind themselves around the host plant pulling itself up by using others for support. It is long lived like a tree (maybe several hundred years) but does not have the trunk, so it comes to a position of dominance by a will to expand rather than through a natural stature. The tiny flowers are curious in that the five petals are joined to form a small cap that is soon pushed off as the stamens ripen beneath. This rejection of the petals illustrates the way that Vine forces its will on those around. The flower is coloured green which like Scleranthus (see p.132) suggests a connection to the heart centre. It is in the heart that the Vine state can become positive. Then the dominant become supportive, the assertive become receptive and the demanding become generous; we become like the Vine itself which provides great riches for mankind in its fruit, the grape.

Locality – Wild and cultivated vines are found throughout the world where the climate is right. Some cultivated Vines grow with difficulty in England but they are not suitable. The photograph on page 149 was taken in Crete.

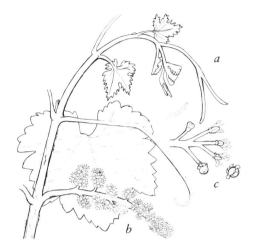 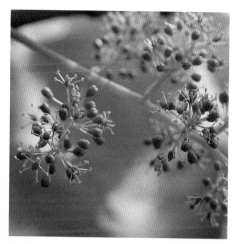

Left: (a) tendrils, (b) flowering stem, (c) flower with petals forced off.   *Right: detail of the flowers.*

Identification – The common grape vine is a perennial, trailing climber. It is usually seen in the cultivated form when it is pruned back to a stubby root stock. In the wild state (sub-species *sylvestris*) stalks can be a considerable length (10-20 m) and on old plants the main stem may be as much as 25 cm in diameter. The leaves are 10-15 cm across with three or five lobes. The flowers form in branched clusters springing from the axil of the leaves. They are small and green with the appearance of closed buds until the petals are forced off by the ripening stamens.

Flowering Period – this varies according to locality. In the Mediterranean it is in early summer: late April to May.

Preparation – Vine is prepared by the sun method (see p.20). The flowering clusters are picked from several different vines when they are in full bloom. This will be when a majority of the flowers are open and beginning to reveal the stamens with pollen. At this time the scent is very apparent. The wild Vine should be used.

WALNUT

We must gain our freedom absolutely and completely, so that all we do, our every action—nay even our every thought—derives its origin in ourselves, thus enabling us to live and give freely of our own accord, and of our own accord alone.

[C.W., 154]

For those who have definite ideals and ambitions in life and are fulfilling them, but on rare occasions are tempted to be led away from their own ideas, aims and work by the enthusiasm, convictions or strong opinions of others.

The remedy gives constancy and protection from outside influences.

[Twelve Healers]

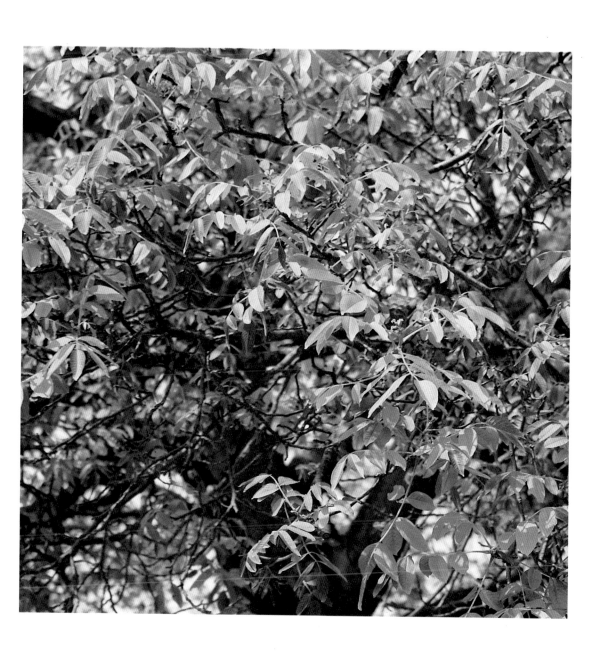

Walnut *Juglans regia*

The idea of companion planting is that certain garden plants co-exist happily together while others are not such good companions. In the wild it is observable that some flowers and trees are inclined to grow together; in part this is because they enjoy the same physical soil conditions but it also indicates a metaphysical relatedness, a linking of their subtle pattern. Walnut trees are quite the reverse. They have an active force that keeps other life forms at bay. It is this quality that makes it the remedy for protection from outside influences. The tree has a fragrant aura that is not unpleasant but it is unattractive to insects, birds and other plants. The smell of the Walnut is particularly strong when the new leaves are breaking bud. The volatile oils evaporate in warm air and at this time it is possible to detect a Walnut tree with your eyes closed! Later in the year it may be necessary to pinch the leaves to sample the scent. As with most plants the activity is strongest earlier in the year when the flowers appear with the new leaves in April and May. This is when the essence is prepared.

The Walnut remedy is not just concerned with protecting our psychological space from interference. It also relates to the process of change and the stages of growth. This is when ties to the past may prevent us from getting on with our new life. Perhaps this process of protecting the new mental pattern is illustrated in the Walnut tree by the nut. It has a soft white kernel formed like the cerebrum of the human brain which is sheltered within a protective fruit. In the positive Walnut state we are able to take up the impression of the new situation without the colouring of old thought patterns. It gives us a kind of immediacy which allows for each new life circumstance to be like a new conception, free from the trammels of the past. The womb-like female Walnut flowers, like all flowers, do conceive afresh each year but no other flower has a fruit that carries so clearly the signature of the human mind. And it is the mind that is influenced in the Walnut condition rather than the feelings.

Locality – Walnut is not a native but has traditionally been planted for the nut as well as for timber. It is often found near to old farmhouses, preferring rich soil and plenty of space in which to grow. Walnuts are mostly found in the southern half of the country where the fruits will ripen.

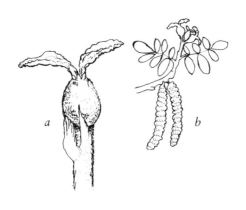 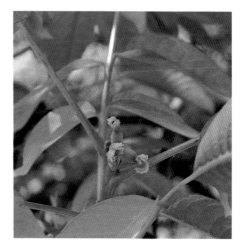

Left: the flowers (a) female, (b) male. **Right:** *detail of the female flowers.*

Identification – Walnuts are deciduous trees of 20-25 m with broad spreading boughs. The bark is generally smooth though old trees are furrowed. The leaves, which are purple green when fresh, are pinnate with between seven and ten leaflets, slightly rounded at the end. The male flowers are fat, pendulous, green catkins. The females are small, green and shaped like a flask (or fig); from the top of the flower two feathery stigmas appear like a tiny rufflet of pale orange-pink which collects the wind-blown pollen. Both flowers appear on the one tree but the males ripen later to ensure cross-pollination from adjacent trees. Because of the scented leaves the Walnut tree cannot be mistaken. Ash, Tree of Heaven and American Black Walnut (*J. nigra*) all have the pinnate leaf though a larger number of leaflets. Black Walnut also has a serrated edge to the leaf (it is not common in Britain). Identification of *J. regia* is easy in April and early May when the leaves appear purple bronze.

Flowering Period – April through to late May.

Preparation – Walnut is prepared by the boiling method (see p.20). Collect from several different trees choosing female flowers, cutting the flowering stems with young leaves so as to fit the saucepan. Some male catkins may be included but it is the female flowers that are important.

WATER VIOLET

AFFIRMATION

...you are learning to stand absolutely alone in the world, gaining the intense joy of complete freedom, and therefore of perfect service to mankind. And when this is realized it is no longer sacrifice but the exquisite joy of helpfulness even under all conditions.

[C.W., 109]

INDICATION

For those who in health or illness like to be alone. Very quiet people, who move about without noise, speak little, and then gently. Very independent, capable and self-reliant. Almost free of the opinions of others. They are aloof, leave people alone and go their own way. Often clever and talented. Their peace and calmness is a blessing to those around them.

[Twelve Healers]

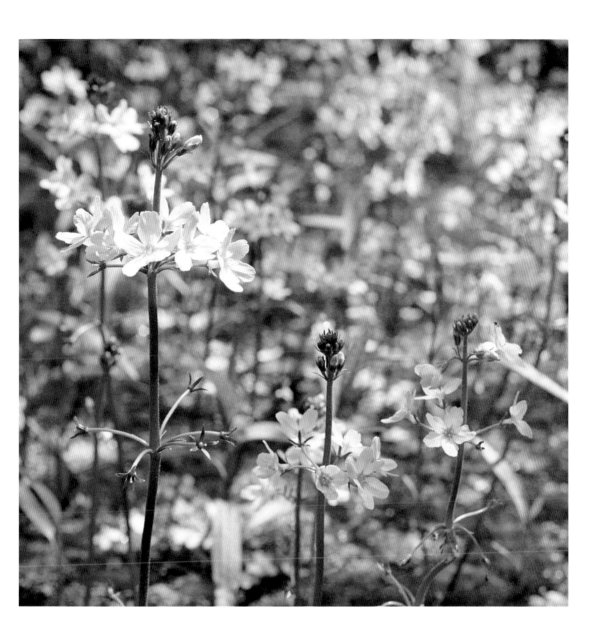

Water Violet *Hottonia palustris*

When Bach found the Water Violet remedy he had been concerned for the health of a friend and knowing her character sought a plant that would help.* He was in that same emotional state himself during the morning. When he saw the Water Violet growing in a stream he knew that it would be right. He placed his hand over the flowers and they brought him to the positive state of the remedy, feeling humble, calm and joyous. We know that the negative Water Violet person is aloof, proud and a little disdainful of life. They like to be alone because other people can be 'vexatious to the spirit'. As it is with the remedy type so it is with the plant. It leads a secluded life, hidden from the public gaze, in the still waters of an undisturbed stream. Even in the 1930s Bach said 'it is comparatively rare, but it is to be found in some of our slow moving crystal brooks and streams' *[C.W., 59]*. Pollution and drainage have destroyed most of them and the Water Violet is now becoming scarce.

Living in water the Water Violet is unapproachable. The dykes where it used to be found are often steep sided and that deters animals just as the aloofness of the person deters other people. Aquatic plants are clearly different in quality (one is minded of the lotus) and perhaps there is something more spiritual about them. The colour of the Water Violet is important too, the pale lilac suggesting a love for humanity and the yellow a clarity of intellect. In early descriptions of Water Violet Bach linked the remedy to the experience of the pain of the world, saying that Water Violet 'will help you to understand that you are being purified through your grief, uplifted to a great ideal, so that you may learn to serve your fellow-men...' *[C.W., 109]*. Although it may be painful it is not through withdrawal but through involvement in life that we find our true being and fulfil our soul's purpose. But the tendency is for the Water Violet to seek seclusion from the onslaught of coarse materialism in our society. As the pressure of our circumstances increases the message of the Water Violet becomes more and more relevant: its retreat from the land is significant in all respects.

Locality – Water Violet grows in drainage ditches and other slow moving water. Many of its traditonal habitats have been destroyed—mechanical ditching has cleared the channels too efficiently, many of the wetland fens have been drained by lowering the water table and various chemicals pollute the dykes. Water Violet is increasingly hard to find but in general terms it grows in southern and eastern counties of England.

* See *Bach Remedy Newsletter*, March 1971; an account by Nora Weeks.

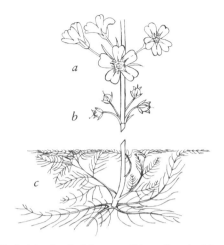 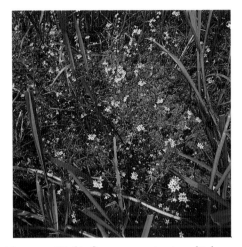

Left: (a) whorl of flowers, (b) seedheads, (c) submerged leaves.   ***Right:*** *flowers growing in a ditch*

Identification – Water Violet is a short-lived perennial aquatic plant. The erect flowering stems grow clear of the water by about 20 cm with the blooms set in whorls. The flowers are simple, five-petalled, like a pale mauve primrose with yellow centres. The feathery leaves remain submerged in the water.

Flowering Period – May and June.

Preparation – Water Violet is prepared by the sun method (see p.20). Pick the individual flowers by the stalk and float them on to the bowl of water.

WHITE CHESTNUT

AFFIRMATION

...the perfect method of learning this is by calm thought and meditation, and by bringing ourselves to such an atmosphere of peace that our Souls are able to speak to us through our conscience and intuition and to guide us according to their wishes.

[C.W., 147]

INDICATION

For those who cannot prevent thoughts, ideas, arguments which they do not desire from entering their minds. Usually at such times when the interest of the moment is not strong enough to keep the mind full.

Thoughts which worry and will remain, or if for a time thrown out, will return. They seem to circle round and round and cause mental torture.

The presence of such unpleasant thoughts drives out peace and interferes with being able to think only of the work or pleasure of the day.

[Twelve Healers]

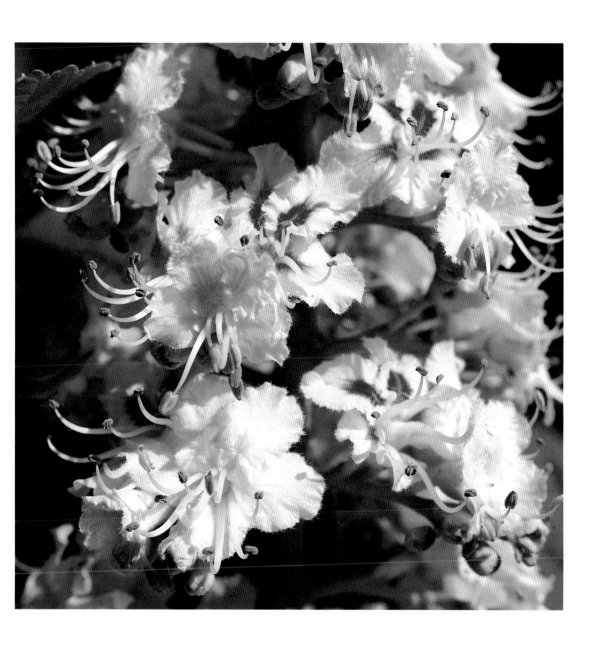

White Chestnut *Aesculus hippocastanum*

The Horse Chestnut tree is a relative newcomer to the English countryside. It arrived from Europe at the beginning of the seventeenth century being a native of the Balkans. Then, as now, it was grown for its attractive blossoms and it has no significant commercial or practical value. Bach called this remedy *White* Chestnut to distinguish it from *Red* Chestnut. However, the trees are closely related in most respects except for colour. It is the action of the colour that is important (see Red Chestnut p.120). Both these trees are concerned with a form of worrying thought. The Red Chestnut having an active colour tends to push that thought externally and express it as a projected worry for the welfare of others. The White Chestnut has a similar pattern of anxiety but it is internal and is expressed as the internal circling pattern of worrying thoughts. These thoughts become mental obsessions that take hold and dominate us. There is no resolution or clarity produced, just an endless train of mental process. The White Chestnut blossom acts to disperse this, replacing it with tranquillity and a proper connection to our inner being; this brings peace. As we reassert the clarity of that calm centre we can view the objective reality of our lives.

As with many of the remedies we can see the positive and negative aspects in the pattern of the tree. Thus the appearance of the flowers on the tree is random and diffused: they are dotted among the leaves as bright lights of activity but without any clear pattern. The individual flowers are not symmetrical and have a crimped and ragged outline. The bark of the tree is broken, irregular and peeling and it adds to the impression of scattered force. So the circular pattern of thoughts is broken, dislocated by the irregularity. Yet, as a whole, the tree is harmonized and balanced. The flowering spikes are like candles, or tapers that burn with the white light of peace. Seen from a distance the tree is decked with bright stars; seen close, the flowers are intense with concentration and yet startling with their pink-throated centres and prominent stamens. Look at the flowers and there is nowhere for the eye to settle, no symmetry except for that of the whole experience.

Locality – Horse Chestnut is tolerant of most soils and conditions but requires full light and space to grow. It is generally seen as a planted tree in parkland and gardens.

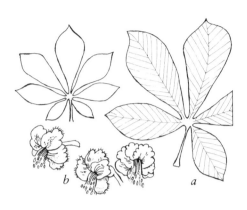 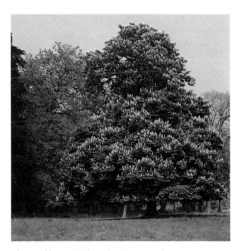

Left: (a) *the palmate leaf,* (b) *single flowers picked from the stalk.*   ***Right:*** *the Horse Chestnut tree.*

Identification – Horse Chestnut is a tree that grows up to 30 m. It grows quickly and probably does not live much beyond 150 years. The trunk is strong and erect with many spreading boughs so the tree has a rounded outline; since cattle eat the leaves up to their head height it often has a flat base. The bark is scaled and breaks into rough squares; the leaves are palmate with five or seven large leaflets. The flowering spikes have blooms on short stalks which are predominantly white with pink, red or yellow centres. The sticky buds and brown conkers are well known (see Chestnut Bud p.50). There is an Indian Horse Chestnut (*A. indica*) with similar flowers but more pointed leaves and smooth grey bark.

Flowering Period – May and June.

Preparation – White Chestnut is prepared by the sun method (see p.20). Pick the individual flowers of the varying colours from several different trees and float them on to the surface of the water.

163

WILD OAT

Let us find the one thing in life that attracts us most and do it. Let that one thing be so part of us that it is as natural as breathing; as natural as it is for the bee to collect honey, and the tree to shed its old leaves in autumn and bring forth new ones in the spring. If we study nature we find that every creature, bird, tree and flower has its definite part to play, its own definite and peculiar work through which it aids and enriches the entire Universe.

[C.W., 97]

INDICATION

Those who have ambitions to do something of prominence in life, who wish to have much experience, and to enjoy all that which is possible for them, to take life to the full.

Their difficulty is to determine what occupation to follow; as although their ambitions are strong, they have no calling which appeals to them above all others.

This may cause delay and dissatisfaction.

[Twelve Healers]

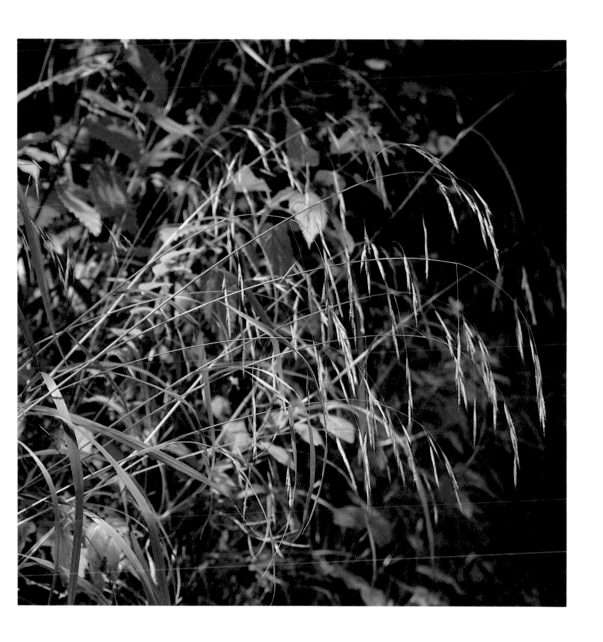

Wild Oat   *Bromus ramosus*

This tall grass is unrelated to the cereal oats and has the undistinguished name of Hairy Brome Grass. Brome comes from the Greek *bromos*, oats. It is one of many varieties of grass which have similar characteristics. Perhaps this is typical of the remedy state where the person has many life possibilities but cannot elect for one clear purpose. It was the last of the *Seven Helpers* and when Bach found it he saw it as being useful as a direction finder that might be needed by anyone. It is a common plant growing on hedge-banks and on the edge of woodland, never forming a strong community but scattered generally. Wild Oat with its tall stem and loose panicle of flowers seems to 'hang around' without a clear direction and pattern of growth. Most of the other grasses form a dense matted covering to the earth and in a spirit of selfless dedication it is their joy to give service. The taller Wild Oat maybe has a deeper purpose but waits in the hedgerow uncertain as to what that is. A hedge is wild ground, a non-specific habitat that has been created by farming enclosures. It is not like the specialized conditions of the water meadow, the chalk downland or a beechwood where other plants may choose to grow. It is a waiting place of unresolved purpose.

In a note that Bach wrote concerning a patient he says of Wild Oat that 'it is for those who are not always in their bodies so cannot see what they are meant to do. It is a state that follows the Clematis state.' Like Clematis (see p.56) the Wild Oat grows with the will to take a firm hold of life. In the negative expression of the remedy this will is not fully effective and then the tendency is to loosen contact with the earth and physical reality. There is a reluctance to define the purpose in our being here on earth and to engage actively in our calling. Wild Oat also relates to Scleranthus, another green flower without petals, which expresses indecision (see p.132). But Scleranthus is earthbound and more concerned with practical problems while the Wild Oat with its swaying long stems has taken to the air. It seeks the purpose of the soul and the true meaning of its life's work.

Locality – Wild Oat grows throughout the country on hedge-banks and along the edge of woodland. It likes a moist soil and prefers a little shade. Look for it where mowers and grazing animals cannot reach on steep banks and among the trees.

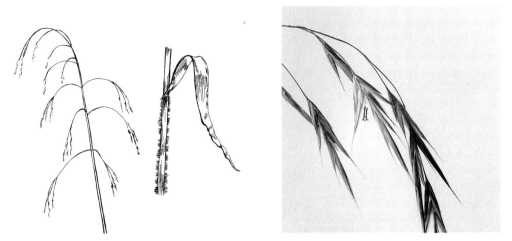

Left: *the panicle of flowers and the hairy stem.* **Right:** *a single flowering stalk.*

Identification – Wild Oat is a very tall grass with a few slender stalks that grow up to 1.5 m or more in height. The leaves are broad blades (15 mm wide) which clasp the stems to form a sheaf which is very hairy. The flowering heads (panicles) are loose like the true oat. Although it is difficult to define a technical identification it should be possible to recognize Wild Oat as different from the other Bromes. The important pointers are the height, the hairs and the appearance of the panicle—see drawing.

Flowering Period – July and August, significantly later than most of the other flowering grasses.

Preparation – Wild Oat is prepared by the sun method (see p.20). When the flower is ready the bracts suddenly open to reveal the rusty brown pollen on the anthers. Pick the flowering ends of the spikelets from many different grasses and float them on to the water.

WILD ROSE

Resignation, which makes one become merely an unobservant passenger on the journey of life, opens the door to untold adverse influences which would never have an opportunity of gaining admittance as long as our daily existence brought with it the spirit and joy of adventure.

[C.W., 149]

Those who without apparently sufficient reason become resigned to all that happens, and just glide through life, take it as it is, without any effort to improve things and find some joy. They have surrendered to the struggle of life without complaint.

[Twelve Healers]

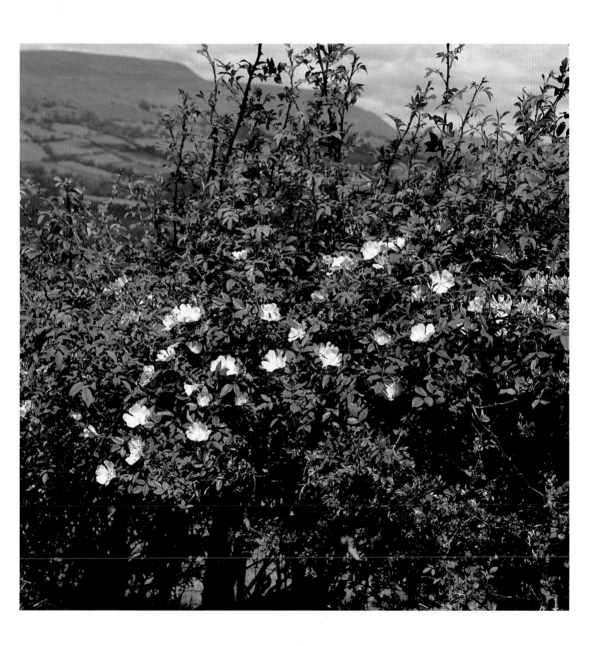

Wild Rose *Rosa canina*

Much of life appears a struggle and in the face of difficulties some of us become resigned to our situation and give up any attempt to improve matters. This kind of resignation does not come through depression or defeat but because we surrender to the forces of inertia. We cannot be bothered. We lose interest in changing and since life is characterized by change we move towards death. When Bach discovered the Wild Rose remedy, which is for this condition, he contrasted it with the Vervain personality (see p.144). The Vervain type goes on fighting and, intolerant of life's shortcomings, they continually try to correct the failings of others. But the Wild Rose people, he said, lack such courage to assert themselves. As Vervain is an over-expression so Wild Rose is an under-expression. This can be seen in the flowers—Vervain's are very small, facing horizontally, while the Wild Rose has flowers that face upwards to the sun, lying open and flat with broad heart-shaped petals. So they absorb more through their surface area and have great strength and vitality to give. The positive of the Wild Rose state has hope and joy so that we start to sing again. But more especially it has determination so that we renew our efforts to live. We feel like getting back to work. Mentally we are reawakened and creative; we become purposeful.

The rose has been cultivated since ancient times. The sweet scent and beauty of the flowers have given it an especial attraction and a symbolism that has always been recognized. In the language of flowers roses speak to the poet, to lovers and to mystics alike. Of course there are many thousands of varieties and each has its particular pattern but it is the simple Dog Rose that Bach chose. It straggles the hedgerows in midsummer, flowering when the sun is at its height. Blushed with pink the Wild Rose adorns the wayside displaying the great desire and love that life has for itself. It is this love for life that is in the positive remedy state. The flower that opens itself completely, basking in the delight of being, calls us to remember that we are as lovers in the daily round of life, awaiting meetings and adventure with a joyful anticipation.

Locality – Wild Rose is a true native rose that grows throughout the country though it is more numerous in the south. It is the common briar of the hedgerow.

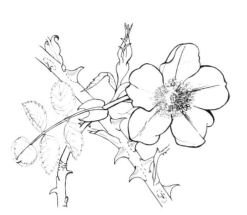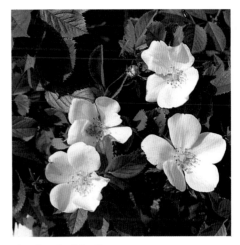

Left: a flowering stalk with thorns, leaf and flower.   *Right: detail of the flowers.*

Identification – The Wild or Dog Rose is a bushy perennial with arched and trailing stems up to about 4m. The curved thorns that possibly resemble a dog's canine tooth are prominent on the otherwise smooth stalks. Leaves are pinnate with five or more usually seven leaflets with serrated edges. The flowers have five heart-shaped petals, large and flat (50mm), either white or pink. The characteristic rosehip appears in autumn. Of the other field roses the Sweet Briar (*R. rubiginosa*) is more heavily scented with many sharp hairs on the stems; Trailing Rose (*R. arvensis*) like *R. stylosa* has a prominent united style in the middle of the flower; the Downy Rose (*R. tormentosa*) which is found mainly on chalk, has furry leaves.

Flowering Period – June and July.

Preparation – Wild Rose is prepared by the boiling method (see p.20). Collect the roses from as many bushes as possible. The flowerheads with a short length of stalk and any leaves should be cut about 15cm in length, so as to fit the saucepan.

WILLOW

We are not all asked to be saints or martyrs or men of renown; to most of us less conspicuous offices are allotted. But we are all expected to understand the joy and adventure of life and to fulfil with cheerfulness the particular piece of work which has been ordained for us by our Divinity.

[C.W., 153]

INDICATION

For those who have suffered adversity or misfortune and find these difficult to accept, without complaint or resentment, as they judge life much by the success which it brings.

They feel that they have not deserved so great a trial, that it was unjust, and they often become embittered.

They often take less interest and less activity in those things of life which they had previously enjoyed.

[Twelve Healers]

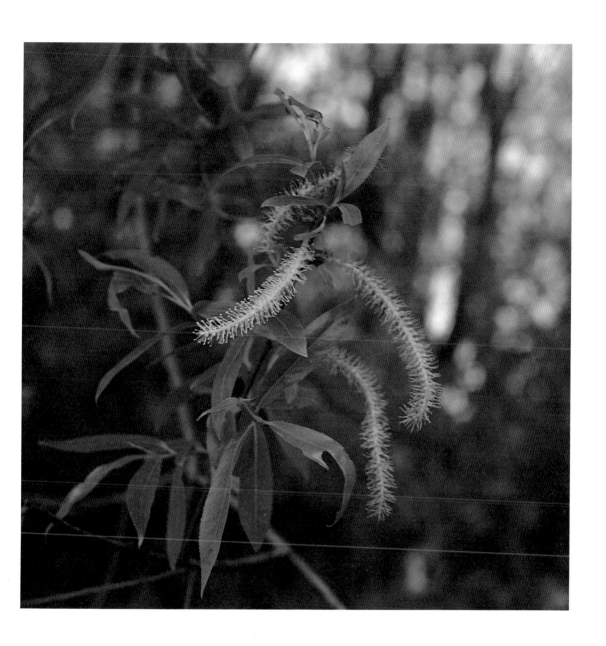

Willow *Salix vitellina*

Just as some animals have been domesticated by man while others remain wild, so plants and trees have been pressed into service wherever they offer a particular use to industry or agriculture. Some plants have quite readily lent themselves to the development of vegetable hybrids (like the cabbage family) while others have remained true to their form but are so used that their pattern is modified. In the case of the Willow tree it remains unchanged but its accepting nature is illustrated by the way that it survives the cruel cutting that it receives. The process of *pollarding*, cutting the branches back to a stump to force new growth, was once widely practised. Every year the vigorous young shoots were taken as wattle for building walls, as withies for basket-making, while other branches were cut in the following years for fencing and as poles. Because the White Willow is flexible and does not snap easily (unlike the Crack Willow) it was ideal for such purposes. It is this flexible tolerance that characterizes the positive Willow state. Since it has been so mistreated as a tree and suffered such abuse it might be turned to bitterness and resentment. Instead it gives of its best with resilient new growth and a constant effort to grow back as a full tree.

Bach's choice of Willow as the remedy for those who complain that they are ill-treated is further illustrated by the way that it grows. Any branch will strike roots without difficulty; cut a Willow pole, drive it into the ground and it will become a tree. Willow has such a will to grow! That is how many of them come to mark field boundaries as we see them today. Its chosen habitat is in wet ground by a river. Here it thrives in rheumatic dampness where other trees may rot or become choked by mosses. As a water lover it is perhaps closest to Water Violet. But while the Water Violet silently grieves for the pain of humanity the Willow (in its negative state) bitterly complains of its own selfish problems. Life is unfair to the Willow types, they feel that they personally deserve better and resent the good fortune of others. They are soured by life. This condition is improved by an effort of positive will and the determination to overcome the difficulties of the situation. The bright golden winter twigs of the *vitellina* Willow emphasize this positive life-affirming quality.

Locality – White Willow trees grow throughout Britain, and the sub-species *S. vitellina* is also found generally. Willows like damp, low-lying land, often lining the banks of rivers and streams.

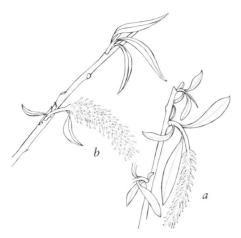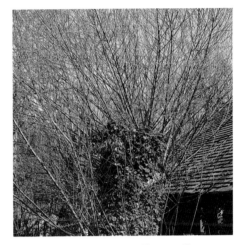

Left: flowers (a) female, (b) male.   **Right:** *the yellow branches of a pollarded 'vitellina' Willow.*

Identification – Willows take several different forms and some care is required to recognize the correct one. *Salix vitellina*, which Bach chose, resembles the White Willow (*S. alba*) in almost all respects. It is a large tree, up to 25 m, with roughly furrowed yellow-green bark. The main trunk is not tall, maybe 3-4 m, as it can branch into several large, spreading boughs. It is often pollarded at this height. The leaves are lanceolate, long and pointed and finely toothed. They have fine white hairs on the underside, unlike the Crack Willow (*S. fragilis*) which has smooth leaves. Male and female flowers appear on different trees: long slightly stiff green catkins. The way to distinguish *S. vitellina* from the White Willow is by the winter twigs which are bright golden yellow, the colour of egg-yolk (hence *vitellina*). The twigs are flexible and do not snap like the Crack Willow. A cross between *S. vitellina* and *S. babylonica*, the Weeping Willow, produced the ornamental Golden Weeping Willow, easily recognized as different because of the drooping twigs.

Flowering Period – during April or May as the leaves unfold.

Preparation – Willow is prepared by the boiling method (see p.20). Male or female catkins are collected from several different trees with about 15 cm of twig and young leaves, so as to fit the saucepan.

Bibliography

There are many books available that illustrate flowers and trees. Some like 'Johns' or 'Keble Martin' are more technical, others, such as the Readers Digest guides, are generalized but probably the more helpful. This list is selected because each book has been worked with and found particularly useful.

Blamey, M. & P. *Flowers of the Countryside*, Collins; 1980
Fitter, R. & A. *Wild Flowers of Britain & N. Europe;* Collins, 1974
Fitter, A. *New Generation Guide to the Wild Flowers of Britain & N. Europe;* Collins, 1987
Forestry Commission, *Know Your Broadleaves;* H.M.S.O., 1968
Grigson, G. *The Englishman's Flora;* Phoenix House, 1958
Grieves, M. *A Modern Herbal;* Cape, 1977
Hyams, E. *The Story of England's Flora;* Kestrel Books, 1979
Johns, Rev. C. A. *Flowers of the Field;* 1899
Keble Martin, W. *The Concise British Flora in Colour;* Rainbird, 1965
Philips, R. *Trees in Britain, Europe & N. America;* Pan Books, 1978
    Wild Flowers of Britain; Pan Books, 1977
Polunin, O. *Trees & Bushes of Britain & Europe;* O.U.P.; 1976
Readers Digest: *Field Guide to Trees & Shrubs of Britain,* 1981
    Field Guide to Wild Flowers of Britain, 1981

BOOKS ON THE FLOWER REMEDIES

Bach, Dr E. *Collected Writings of Edward Bach*, Bach Educational Programme; 1987
    The Twelve Healers & Other Remedies, C.W. Daniel; 1936
Barnard, J. *A Guide to the Bach Flower Remedies*, C.W. Daniel; 1979
    Patterns of Life Force, Bach Educational Programme; 1987
Chancellor, P.M. *Handbook of the Bach Flower Remedies,* C.W. Daniel; 1971
Scheffer, M. *Bach Flower Therapy*, Thorsons; 1986
Vlamis, G. *Flowers to the Rescue*, Thorsons; 1986
Weeks, N. *The Medical Discoveries of Edward Bach Physician*, C.W. Daniel; 1973
Weeks, N. & Bullen, V. *The Bach Flower Remedies, Illustrations and Preparation,*
                                      C.W. Daniel; 1964